Dr. Jensen's
GUIDE TO DIET AND
DETOXIFICATION

Dr. Jensen's
GUIDE TO DIET AND DETOXIFICATION

Bernard Jensen, D.C., Ph.D.
Clinical Nutritionist

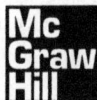

Mc Graw Hill

New York   Chicago   San Francisco   Lisbon   London   Madrid   Mexico City
Milan   New Delhi   San Juan   Seoul   Singapore   Sydney   Toronto

The *McGraw·Hill* Companies

Library of Congress Cataloging-in-Publication Data

Jensen, Bernard, 1908–.
  [Guide to diet and detoxification]
  Dr. Jensen's guide to diet and detoxification / Bernard Jensen.
       p.   cm.
  Includes index.
  ISBN 0-658-00275-9
     1. Nutrition.   2. Detoxification (Health)   I. Title: Doctor Jensen's guide to diet
  and detoxification.   II. Title.

  RA784.5 .J46   2000
  615.8'54—dc21   00-43450

10 11 12 13 14 15 16 17 18 19 20 21 22 23 24 25 26   WFR/WFR 0

ISBN 978-0-07-183676-0

Design by Andrea Reider
Illustration, page 5, by Elizabeth Weadon Massari
Illustrations, pages 41–42, by Ilene Robinette Studio

McGraw-Hill books are available at special quantity discounts to use as premiums and sales promotions or for use in corporate training programs. To contact a representative, please visit the Contact Us pages at www.mhprofessional.com.

The purpose of this book is to educate. It is sold with the understanding that the publisher and author shall have neither liability nor responsibility for any injury caused or alleged to be caused directly or indirectly by the information contained in this book. While every effort has been made to ensure its accuracy, the book's contents should not be construed as medical advice. Each person's health needs are unique. To obtain recommendations appropriate to your particular situation, please consult a qualified health care provider.

This book is printed on acid-free paper.

It has been my great pleasure to incorporate the nature care approach to healing into my sixty years of practice. I am very grateful to those patients who followed by teachings in this healing method and proved its effectiveness. I want to acknowledge with thanks all those patients who have had the fortitude to stick with me and trust me as they experienced many elimination processes and healing crises on the path to the better health they were seeking. . . .

—Bernard Jensen, D.C., Ph.D.

"Seek not to learn, but to think. Seek not to accept what is told you, but to question. . . . It is a good student who will question what is taught him. . . . And it is a good professor who, if he is not sure of his ground, will link arms with the student and say, 'Let us go and find out.' . . ."

"Remember that fifteen units of study a semester may eventually lead to a degree, but not necessarily to a real education. . . . You will find that the mind is not a pail to fill, but a dynamo to start working."

—From a speech by a university president
to a gathering of students.

OTHER KEATS TITLES BY DR. BERNARD JENSEN:

Dr. Jensen's Juicing Therapy
Dr. Jensen's Nutrition Handbook
Dr. Jensen's Guide to Body Chemistry & Nutrition

CONTENTS

INTRODUCTION

*Nature's creative power exceeds man's
inclination to destroy.*

I t should be noted that 80 percent of all diseases in the United States are of a chronic
nature. People develop chronic diseases over a period of years, as
will be explained later.

I would like to give first a briefing on how my treatments
work. To overcome a chronic disease requires right living, good
food, and an elimination and detoxification program. In almost
all cases, I start with detoxification. I like my patients, new and
old, to be familiar with elimination diets, detoxification, the
reversal process, and the healing crisis—and to have a clear
understanding of them.

CHAPTER 1

DEATH BEGINS
IN THE COLON

The expression "Death begins in the colon" apparently originated with the Nobel prize–winning Russian biologist Elie Metchnikoff (1845–1916) during his later years of laboratory research at the Pasteur Institute in Paris. While studying the flora of the human intestine, he became convinced that aging and death were gradually caused by the destructive influence on the body by toxic metabolic by-products of bowel bacteria. He advocated the use of fermented milk products rich in beneficial microorganisms, such as *Lactobacillus acidophilus,* to crowd out the harmful bacteria and reduce their negative influence on health and aging processes. The fame that followed his 1908 Nobel prize (in physiology, shared with Paul Erlich), together with many other prestigious awards and honors by other institutions, caused his opinion about the link between bowel toxins and health to be broadly accepted by allopathic physicians and natural cure doctors alike, as well as the general public in Europe and North America.

Among those persons greatly influenced by Metchnikoff were Sir Arbuthnot Lane, M.D. (1856–1943), physician to the royal family of Great Britain, and John Harvey Kellogg, M.D. (1852–1943), surgeon and founder of the famed Battle Creek Sanitarium. Both doctors emphasized the importance of bowel cleanliness to good health and longevity and both condemned toxemia of the bowel as the basic cause of most disease.

Dr. Lane claimed to have cured conditions such as arthritis, asthma, and goiter by surgically removing certain sections of the bowel. During the last twenty-five years of his life, Dr. Lane turned from surgery to nutrition as the most effective antidote to bowel toxemia. He said, "All maladies are due to the lack of certain food principles, such as mineral salts or vitamins, or to the absence of the normal defenses of the body, such as the natural protective flora. When this occurs, toxic bacteria invade the lower alimentary canal, and the poisons thus generated pollute the bloodstream and gradually deteriorate and destroy every tissue, gland, and organ of the body."

Dr. John Harvey Kellogg, a vegetarian, believed that the main culprit in bowel toxemia was meat eating and stated, "The putrefactive changes which recur in the undigested residues of flesh foods were to blame for 90 percent of all illness." According to Josh Clark, one of Kellogg's biographers, "Kellogg's influence and enthusiasm made the bowel not only an acceptable subject of polite conversation, but a national obsession." In other words, the trend toward better nutrition and bowel care was moving in the direction of improved health through greater harmony between man and nature during at least the first quarter of the twentieth century.

State of the art research on intestinal toxemia in more recent years is confirming the basic discoveries of the late nineteenth and early twentieth centuries.

According to a recent news release by the International Foundation for Functional Gastrointestinal Disorders, millions of people of all ages, up to 20 percent of the total population—men, women, and children—are afflicted with gastrointestinal disorders. Irritable bowel syndrome (IBS) is responsible for more absenteeism from work than any other affliction except the common cold. Indigestion, sometimes involving bad food or pathogens, is also near the top of the list of gastrointestinal problems. An article published in the October 1998 issue of the English medical journal *The Lancet* has linked food fermentation or toxins released during fermentation with IBS. An enterotoxin from bacteria named *bacteroides fragilis* has been recently linked with inflammatory bowel disease (IBD), according to a March–April 2000 article in the journal *Emerging Infectious Diseases.* Other viruses and bacteria are known to be involved in IBD and IBD relapses following dormant phases of the disease. The article pointed out that the adult colon is a "complex ecosystem of approximately five hundred species of . . . microorganisms," despite the fact that the intestine of a newborn lacks organisms of any kind.

We need to be aware that the bowel environment inside each of us is determined by a combination of factors. The relative constitutional strength or weakness of our gastrointestinal system is one factor. The climate, altitude, vegetation, and degree of urbanization (noise, smog, and encounters with people) are other factors. What we take into our lungs and through our skin influences the bowel. The great influence, however, is what goes into our mouth, stomach, and bowel—and, at least for some people, this might include a host of body pollutants—drugs, alcohol, chemical food additives, pesticide residues, foods deficient in nutrients, foods changed either physically or chemically by processing, and soil contaminants. The detoxification capability of our liver and immune system helps determine what toxins manage to get from the bowel into the circulating blood. The level of physical activity we get into day by day, including exercise, influences the bowel environment directly but also through the influence of activities on our oxygen intake, metabolic level, lymph system efficiency, and blood circulation. Obviously, these factors combine in different ways to form a great variety of bowel environments, which will greatly influence the kinds of organisms—good and bad—that live and thrive in our bowels.

Worldwide, the greatest threat to life and health is parasites—mostly bowel parasites. Not heart disease, cancer, or dysentery, but parasites. And sometimes the greatest threat is not from the parasites themselves but from their metabolic waste products, which can be extremely toxic.

One of the best descriptions I've found of the chemical contents of the bowel (excluding microorganisms) is from a report published in the *World Iridology Fellowship Journal,* December 1974, through the courtesy of George Lachnicht Jr., D.C. I am reproducing it here as in the original report.

> The following report, *Discussion of Alimentary Toxemia,* was given before the Royal Society of Medicine of Great Britain:
> Recently, the subject of alimentary toxemia (see fig. 1.1) was discussed in London before the Royal Society of Medicine by fifty-seven of the leading physicians of Great Britain. Among the speakers were eminent surgeons, physicians, and specialists in the various branches of medicine. The following is a list of the various poisons of alimentary intestinal toxemia noted by the several speakers: Indol, skatol, phenol, cresol, indican, hydrogen sulfide, ammonia, histidine, urobilin, methylmercaptan, tetramerthylendiamin, pentamethylendiamine, putrescine, cadaverine, neurine, choline, muscarine, butyric acid, beraimidazzolethylamine, methylgandiamine, ptomarropine, botulin, tyramine, agamatine, trypto-

phan, sepsin, idolethylamine, and sulpherroglobine. Of these thirty-six poisons just mentioned, several are highly active, producing most profound effects, and in very small quantities. In cases of alimentary toxemia, some one or several of these poisons is constantly bathing the delicate body cells and setting up changes that finally result in a grave disease.

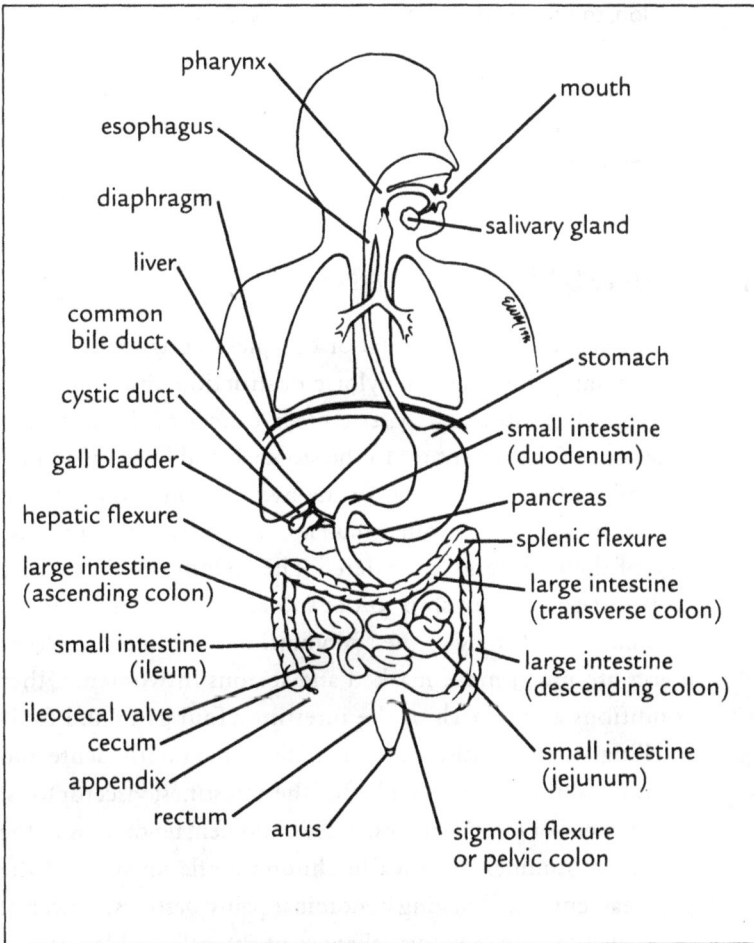

Figure 1.1. **The alimentary canal, thirty feet in length, consists of the mouth, pharynx, esophagus, and the organs of digestion—the stomach, and the small and large intestines.**

It should be understood that these findings are not mere theories, but are the results of demonstration in actual practice by eminent physicians. Of course, it is not claimed that alimentary toxemia is the only cause of all the symptoms and diseases named; although, of many, it may be the sole or principal cause, some of them due to other causes as well. In the following summary, the various symptoms and disorders mentioned in the discussion in London, to which reference has been made above, are grouped and classified.

The conditions found in the following organs or systems substituted are or can be caused by toxic chemicals in the bowel, as previously listed.

THE DIGESTIVE ORGANS

Duodenal ulcer causes partial or complete obstruction of the duodenum: pyloric spasm, pyloric obstruction, distension and dilation of the stomach, gastric ulcer, cancer of the stomach, adhesions of the omentum to the stomach and liver, inflammation of the liver, and cancer of the liver. The muscular wall of the intestines as well as other muscles, atrophies, so that the passage of their contents is hindered. The abdominal viscera lose their normal relationship to the spine and to each other, on account of weakening of the abdominal muscles; these displacements are much more marked and serious in women. Other conditions are: catarrh of the intestines; foul gases and foul-smelling stools; colitis; acute enteritis; appendicitis, acute and chronic; adhesions and "kinks" of the intestines; visceroptosis; enlargement of the spleen; distended abdomen; tenderness of the abdomen; summer diarrhea in children; inflammation of the pancreas; chronic dragging abdominal pains; gastritis; cancer of the pancreas; inflammatory changes of the gall bladder; cancer of the gall bladder; gallstones; degeneration of the liver; cirrhosis of the liver; infection of the gums and decay of the teeth; and ulcers in the mouth and pharynx.

THE HEART AND BLOOD VESSELS

Wasting and weakening of the heart muscles; microbic cyamosis from breaking up of blood cells; fatty degeneration of the heart; endocarditis, myocarditis; subnormal blood pressure; enlargement of the heart; the dilatation of the aorta; high blood pressure; arteriosclerosis; permanent dilation of the arteries. Dr. W. Bezley says, "There are but a few phases of cardiovascular trouble (disease of heart and blood vessels) with which disorder of some part of the alimentary tract is not causatively associated."

THE NERVOUS SYSTEM

Headaches of various kinds—frontal, occipital, temporal, dull or intense, hemicranic; headache of a character to lead to a mistaken diagnosis of brain tumor. Dr. Lane tells of a case where a surgeon had proposed an operation for the removal of a tumor from the frontal lobe of the brain; the headaches were wholly resolved by removing a section of the colon. Other nerve problems related to the colon included acute neuralgia pains in the legs; neuritis; twitching of the eyes and of muscles of the face, arms, legs, etc.; disturbances of the nervous system from simple headaches to absolute collapse; mental and physical depression; insomnia; paralysis; chronic fatigue; morbid introspection; melancholia, mania; difficulty in mental concentration; insanity and delirium.

THE EYES

Degenerative changes in the eye, inflammation of the lens, inflammation of the optic nerve, hardening of the lens, sclerotitis, sclerokeratitis, iritis, iridocyclitis, cataract, recurrent hemorrhage in the retina, eye dull and heavy.

THE SKIN

Formation of wrinkles; thin, inelastic, starchy skin; pigmentations of the skin—yellow, brown, slate-black, blue; muddy complexion;

thickening of the skin of the back—sores and boils; pemphigus; pruritus; herpes; eczema; dermatitis; lupus erythematosus; acne rosacea; cold, clammy extremities; dark circles under the eyes; seborrhea; psoriasis; pityriasis, alopecia, lichen; planus; jaundice.

An infinitesimal amount of toxin may suffice to cause skin eruption.

THE MUSCLES AND JOINTS

Degeneration of the muscles: Muscles waste and become soft and in advanced cases tear easily. In young life, the muscular debility produces the deformities which are called dorsal excurvation, or round shoulders; lateral curvature; flat-foot; and knock-knee. Weakness of abdominal muscles causes accumulation of feces in the pelvic colon, which renders evacuation of contents more and more difficult. Prominence of bones; rheumatic pains simulating sciatica and lumbago; various muscular pains; muscular rheumatism; arthritis deformities; synovitis; rickets; arthritis, acute and chronic. Tubercles and rheumatoid arthritis are the direct result of intestinal intoxication. Dr. Lane says, "I do not believe it is possible for either of these diseases to obtain a foothold except in the presence of stasis."

GENITOURINARY AND REPRODUCTIVE ORGANS

Various displacements, distortion, and disease of the uterus; change in the whole contour of woman; fibrosis of breast; wasting of breasts; induration of breasts; subacute and chronic mastitis; cancer of breast; metritia and endometritis; infection of bladder especially in women; frequent urination; albuminuria; acute nephritis; movable kidney; floating kidney. Dr. Lane goes so far as to say, "Autointoxication plays so large a part in the development of disease of the female genitourinary apparatus, that they may be regarded by the gynecologist as a product of intestinal stasis."

GENERAL DISORDERS AND DISTURBANCES OF NUTRITION

Degeneration of the organs of elimination, especially the liver, kidneys (Bright's disease), and spleen; pernicious anemia; lowered resistance to infection of all kinds; premature senile decay; retardation of growth in children, accompanied by mental irritability and muscular fatigue; adenoids; enlarged tonsils; enlarged thyroid (goiter); various tumors and hypothyroid; Raynaud's disease. In those who apparently suffer no harm from constipation during a long series of years there is, perhaps, a partial immunity established. The writer has long believed that such an immunity is sometimes established in the very obstinate constipation which accompanies absolute fasting because of the cleansing of the tongue and reappearance of appetite which often occurs at the end of the second or third week of the fast, a phenomenon very like that which appears in typhoid fever and other continued fevers. It must not be supposed, however, that even the establishment of so-called immunity ensures the body against all injury. The labor of eliminating an enormous amount of virulent toxins, which falls upon the kidneys, damages the renal tissues and produces premature failure of these essential organs. Any process which develops toxins within the body is a menace to the life of the tissues and should be suppressed as far as possible, and as quickly as possible.

The fact that symptoms of poisoning resulting from constipation do not appear at once is no evidence that injury is not done. Dr. William Hunter in the course of the London discussion remarked that the fact that chronic constipation "might exist in certain individuals as an almost permanent condition without apparently causing ill health is due solely to the power and protective action of the liver. It is not any evidence of the comparative harmlessness of constipation per se, but only evidence that some individuals possess the cecum and the colon of an ox, with the liver of a pig, capable of doing any amount of distoxication." In the face of such an array of evidence backed up by authority of nearly sixty eminent English physicians—and many hundreds of other English, U.S., German, and French physicians whose names might be added—it is no longer possible to ignore the importance of alimentary toxemia or autointoxication as a fact in the production of disease. To no other single cause is it possible to attribute one-tenth as many various and widely diverse disorders. It may be said that almost every chronic disease known is directly or indirectly due to the influence of bacterial poisons absorbed from the intestine. The colon may be justly looked upon as a veritable Pandora's box, out of which come more human misery and suffering, mental and moral, as well as physical, than from any other known source.

The colon is a sewage system, but by neglect and abuse it becomes a cesspool. When it is clean and normal, we are well and happy; let it stagnate, and it will distill the poisons of decay, fermentation, and putrefaction into the blood, poisoning the brain and nervous system so that we become mentally depressed and irritable; it will poison the heart so that we are weak and listless; poison the lungs so that the breath is foul; poison the digestive organs so that we are distressed and bloated; and poison the blood so that the skin is sallow and unhealthy. In short, every organ of the body is poisoned, and we age prematurely, look and feel old, the joints are stiff and painful, neuritis, dull eyes, and a sluggish brain overtake us; the pleasure of living is gone.

The preceding information should impress you with the vital importance of bowel regularity to you and every member of your family.

I would like to point out that toxins in the body, whether generated from within, as in autointoxication, or without, as from drugs, caffeine, contaminated drinking water, chemicals in food products, polluted air, or other sources, have a devastating effect on the natural defenses of the body. In this way, toxins produce a disease-vulnerable body environment. Even though body toxins may not be the causes of all diseases, they prepare the body to accept many illnesses and diseases that would not have flourished or even gained a foothold in a healthy body.

CHAPTER 2

AUTOINTOXICATION

A utointoxication is defined as the poisoning of the body, or some part of the body, by toxic matter generated therein.

The following excerpt appeared in the *World Iridology Fellowship Journal* of December 1974, on the subject of autointoxication resulting from intestinal putrefaction and the finding of *indican*—a by-product of putrefaction—in urine:

> Stedman's Medical Dictionary: Indican—the mother substance of indigo-blue, a yellowish or colorless syrupy glucoside; or indoxyl sulphate, a substance found in the sweat and in variable amounts in urine.
>
> Indicanuria: The presence in excess in the urine of indican, derived from indole produced in protein putrefaction in the intestine and in putrefactive changes elsewhere. (Indican = Indoxyl potassium sulphate.) In gallstone attacks, in hyperchlorhydria, in recurring appendicitis, in wasting diseases, in peritonitis, and in empyema, it is usually present. In a few cases it is constant.
>
> The enzymes in and produced by microorganisms in the intestine break down some of the undigested polysaccharides, proteins, and other complex compounds. Comment has been made that the

end products from carbohydrate breakdown are usually innocuous, whereas many of the compounds resulting from the decomposition of protein are toxic. The latter fact has given rise to the assumption that when the rate of production and absorption of these products is increased above normal, as in constipation, a condition of autointoxication is produced, which is characterized by malaise, headache, irritability, and other symptoms.

It should be borne in mind that no trace of indican may, or may not, be indicative of the absence of putrefaction. In the absence of putrefaction, a negative reading would be expected, but a single test cannot be relied upon. Experience has shown that a restored efficiency of the manifold eliminative processes may increase excretion of indican, and this would be indicative of retention of the products of putrefaction previously.

Apart from internal processes that lead to autointoxication, there are numerous environmental toxins that people are exposed to. Although this is not the place for a comprehensive listing, this chapter would not be complete without a clear warning of the dangers that beset us as by-products of our postindustrial, high-tech contamination of our surroundings, most particular in urban areas of the country.

ENVIRONMENTAL TOXINS

Heavy Metals

Although cleanup of lead, mercury, and arsenic has been extensive in the past five decades, we still encounter these toxic substances. Cadmium, which comes from cigarette smoke, batteries, hot water pipes, and zinc processing plants, is still widespread and just as dangerous as lead. I can't think of a metal that isn't toxic at high levels of exposure, but the problem with the heavy metals is that they aren't excreted adequately in the urine, and even trace amounts can create health problems. Dr. Henry A. Schroeder has pointed out, "There are thousands of examples of toxicity from exposure of workers to metals and metal dusts." Toxicity from nickel, selenium, and chromium is well documented, yet all three of these metals are essential nutrients in trace amounts. Mental retardation, cancer, lung diseases, nerve damage, skin problems, gastrointestinal damage, and kidney failure are a few of the conditions that metal poisoning can cause.

Industrial Toxins

Benzene, dyes, polychlorinated biphenyls, sulfur dioxide, nitrogen dioxide, asbestos, sodium hydroxide, perchloroethylene, methylene chloride, trichlorethylene, and thousands of other industrial toxins are present in our environment. They come from smoke, machine exhausts, strong chemicals used in industrial processes, manufacturing waste by-products, burning coal, gasoline, diesel fuel, and other sources, resulting in cancer, birth defects, lung diseases, kidney and heart problems, and so forth. We are exposed to industrial toxins primarily in our air and water. Coal miners, for example, get black lung disease from breathing in coal dust.

Drinking Water

For many years, most of us thought that chlorination of our drinking water would get rid of germs and amoebas, but in the last thirty years or so, chemists have found that chlorine in treated public water supplies may combine with organic materials to produce chloramines, which cause cancer. Chlorine is claimed to be associated with a 20 to 40 percent increase in colorectal cancer. Thousands of public water supplies as of this date do not meet the purity standards the federal government has established. *E. coli,* a common bacteria wherever animals are found, is a common contaminant of wells. Surface water is often polluted by sewage, manufacturing waste chemicals, acid rain, and organic debris. Underground water becomes contaminated with arsenic, nitrates, phosphates, ether, and radioactive chemicals. I use reverse osmosis water, even though my well water is still clean.

Tobacco Smoke

One government report I read said that there were more than four thousand chemicals in tobacco, including twelve known to cause cancer. The chemicals in cigarettes include nicotine, methanol, cadmium, acetaldehyde, lead, arsenic, formaldehyde, hydrazine, polonium, benzopyrene, carbon monoxide, and others. Smoking is the primary cause of bronchitis and many types of cancer. Cigarette companies in recent years have been held responsible in the courts for smoking-related health problems among their customers and have had to pay out billions of dollars. I believe that cigarettes are finally on their way out.

Air Pollution

I've been told that even the ancient Romans complained of irritating smoke in the air on some occasions. But if you've ever been in Los Angeles when the air was so brown you could hardly see the building across the street, your experience was much more dangerous, I believe, than that of the Romans. Modern air pollution in the United States varies from area to area. In urban locations, it is made up of auto exhaust emissions, industrial pollutants, particulate matter (such as dust and pollens), gases, soot, smoke, and acid rain. (When acid rain lands in lakes and streams, it turns into sulfuric acid and nitrous or nitric acid, deadly to fish, frogs, and other water creatures. Gases include carbon monoxide, ozone, nitrogen oxides, sulfur dioxide, and volatile organic compounds. Particulate matter includes plant spores, dust and sand particles, and smoke and soot from fires. Industrial pollutants have been covered, but we also need to know that indoor pollutants can be harmful to our health. Office machines, such as typewriters, copy machines, computers, fax machines and printers, and other sources, such as cleaning chemicals, carpets, and padded chairs, may emit a variety of chemical odors and gases that can make people sick.

DIETARY TOXINS

All the preceding described toxins added to the toxins our bodies produce internally mean that the health risk is much higher now for most of us than it was a hundred years ago. In turn, this means it is of vital importance that we learn how to keep our bodies strong and clean. We must pay special attention to eating the right foods and keeping our elimination organs in good condition.

Consider the average person walking down the street . . . chances are he or she is at least half sick. We think of the man who fell out of a twenty-story window. As he passed the second story window, he remarked, "Well, I'm all right so far!" So it is with people living dangerously, partaking of foods that put them at risk for toxemia. They may be "all right so far," but how long will it last?

Unfortunately, many people living dangerously do not realize what they are doing. They continue to drink alcoholic beverages or beverages compromised with toxic chemical additives, smoke tobacco, overeat, and partake of foods difficult to digest, such as white bread or foods containing white sugar. They just do not understand the effects of bad food, smoking, and drinking habits. They do not know, for instance, that a shortage of natural, fresh foods in the diet will create a shortage of enzymes and a corresponding increase in the work of the enzyme-producing glands.

For example, a food such as papaya has a considerable quantity of enzymes. By eating this food and other foods containing enzymes, we can avoid overworking the pancreas. The pancreas produces juices needed in digestion. It also produces insulin, needed to control blood sugar. Insufficient ingestion of natural foods, combined with excessive use of foods requiring large amounts of pancreatic secretions, such as white bread and sugar, causes the pancreas to work overtime and to become disabled and underproduce the necessary juices. Insufficient enzymes are said to cause degenerative disease.

Most people know the effects of tobacco on the system. Since the 1964 Surgeon General's Report on Smoking and Health, many Americans have become aware of the connection between smoking and cancer. As Dr. Melchior T. Dikkers has pointed out in his book *Unintentional Suicide,* nicotine and chemicals in tobacco cause the mucous membranes to become chronically inflamed and, consequently, more easily penetrated by toxic chemical gases in the air. This is a direct causative factor in the production of cancer.

People also now know that alcohol destroys important nutrients, leading to vitamin deficiencies and mineral imbalances. There is particularly a shortage created in Vitamin B_1 (thiamine) and nicotinic acid (niacin). In addition, autopsies reveal that the brain of the alcoholic becomes dehydrated and functionally impaired. Alcohol slows down reflex actions, perception, judgment, and speech. Eyesight suffers and muscular coordination is greatly reduced.

Autointoxication is self-poisoning . . . which is slow suicide. When done through ignorance, it is unintentional suicide. When done because of stubbornness, it is intentional suicide. Life can and should be sweet and wonderful.

⚅ Alfalfa

One of the best natural supplements I have found to help the bowel overcome slowed bowel activity due to inherent weaknesses and poor bowel muscle tone is alfalfa tablets. Alfalfa is a very effective remedy for excessively slow bowel transit time. High-fiber supplements and foods high in fiber (such as alfalfa, oat bran, wheat bran, rice bran, and legumes) give the weakened bowel tissue something to push against, and the bowel wall musculature becomes stronger. The chlorophyll found in alfalfa tablets helps to nourish the friendly bacteria, gets rid of odorous gases, and nourishes the beneficial intestinal flora, including the friendly *acidophilus* bacteria. I recommend taking four alfalfa tablets along with each meal. Crack them once before swallowing them. Take them right along with the meal and in between bites of food, as you desire.

LAXATIVES

As a rule, I do not believe in laxatives. Laxatives are usually of an irritable nature, and the body wants to get rid of this irritation and produces an increased peristaltic action to get rid of the impacted material. There are times when a laxative can be used to a good advantage, but it should be of a temporary nature. If you become dependent on laxatives, your bowel will lose its tone and become even more vulnerable to putrefaction, parasites, and injury from toxins.

CHAPTER 3

ELIMINATION DIETS

The purpose of elimination diets is to stimulate the body to release and get rid of toxic wastes, which are usually settled in the fatty tissues; the inherently weak tissues, glands, and organs; lymphatic tissue; and along the bowel walls, especially that of the colon. Elimination diets are what I call "one-sided" diets. Unlike a balanced diet, they are not meant to build and repair tissue along with eliminating unwanted substances from the body.

For your own protection, I advise that you consult your doctor when you intend to use an elimination diet or fasting procedure. It is best to be under the supervision of a doctor or nutritionist for any elimination diet or procedure lasting more than three days, especially if you have any chronic diseases or are over fifty years of age.

ELEVEN-DAY ELIMINATION REGIMEN

I want you to know that there are many procedures we can follow in detoxifying the body. Most people do not drink enough water, eat enough fiber foods, or get enough exercise to prevent bowel stasis and clogged lymph systems, so the body's natural and normal means of ridding itself of toxins is not adequately taken advantage of. There is no great secret to elimination diets and procedures. By using less food, more liquids, simpler foods, and simple food combinations, we simply make it easier for the body to do what it should do naturally.

In outline, our plan for the eleven-day regimen is to begin with water and juices for the first three days; graduating to a diet of fruits, juices, and water for the next two days; then six days on citrus and other fruits, salads, broth, and steamed vegetables. I want you to take a hot bath before going to bed each night.

Gather the foods you will need in advance. They should include lots of fruits and vegetables.

The fruits you may select from are citrus, grapes, melons, tomatoes, pears, peaches, plums, and other fruit in season. Reconstituted dried (unsulfured if available) fruits, such as prunes, figs, apricots, and peaches, may be used. To reconstitute the dried fruit, cover with water in a saucepan, bring to a boil, and let soak overnight. Salads should be garden salads (avoid iceberg lettuce) made with fresh leaf lettuce, sprouts, raw spinach, radishes, celery, green onions, cucumber, raw zucchini, tomatoes, and parsley. A little raw shredded parsnip, carrot, or beet may be sprinkled on top. If you can take the salad without dressing, that would be best. If you need to use dressing, use it sparingly—no more than a tablespoon or two. The last six days you may steam fresh vegetables, such as broccoli, carrots, peas, squash, corn, cauliflower, and snow peas.

Vital broth is an important part of this regimen, and here is my recipe:

VITAL BROTH RECIPE

½ cup carrot tops   *2 cups celery tops*

2 cups potato peelings   *1 teaspoon vegetable*

(½-inch thick)   *broth powder*

2 cups beet tops   *2 quarts distilled water*

3 cups celery stalk   *(Add onion, if desired, for flavor)*

Finely chop first five ingredients, combine with vegetable broth powder and water in pan, bring to a boil slowly, simmer 20 minutes, strain, and use only the broth.

Before I present the schedule for the Eleven-Day Elimination Regimen, I want you to be prepared to use enemas for the first four or five days if you are not having bowel movements. It is not unusual for bowel movements to stop when you cut back on the amount of food you are taking. You may want to take a nap or rest every afternoon of the eleven days. Drink two or three quarts of water each day—eight to twelve 8-ounce glasses per day (one every hour or so) in addition to juices. When you get to the sixth day, eat slowly so that you don't overeat.

Schedule

Days 1 to 3. To start your day, drink two 8-ounce glasses of water. After a half hour to an hour, have your first glass of grapefruit or orange juice, and continue drinking a glass every four hours. The reason I want you to use citrus juice is because it stirs up acids and toxins better than any other juice, and the water helps carry this unwanted material off. Remember to drink a glass of water every hour or so until you've had eight to twelve glasses. Take a hot bath before bed.

Days 4 and 5. Drink two 8-ounce glasses of water upon rising. For meals, eat fruit only, breakfast, lunch, and dinner. You may also drink juice between meals. Be sure you drink six to ten more glasses of water before going to bed. Take a hot bath each night.

Days 6 to 11. Drink two 8-ounce glasses of water after you wake up. For breakfast, take only citrus fruit. Between breakfast and lunch, you may snack on a non-citrus fruit. For lunch, have a garden salad with three to six different vegetables and two cups of vital broth. For dinner, have two or three lightly steamed vegetables and two cups of vital broth. You may use a little sea salt if you have it, or sprinkle a little vegetable broth powder on your veggies and broth for taste. Take a hot bath each night.

For your own good, follow this elimination regimen to the letter. If you make it easier for yourself by adding other foods or different foods, you will interfere with the detoxification process, and the cleansing will not be as thorough as it could have been.

Keep in mind that this Eleven-Day Elimination Regimen can be used as a means of entry into a way of right living. Ultimately, the best way to avoid the buildup of toxins in your body is to change from your old way of living and begin a whole new lifestyle.

If you are not able or willing to make the changes you know you should make, you can still use this elimination regimen three times a year or so. It will help with weight control, with reducing the pain and stiffness in joints, with skin that is breaking out, and with chronic constipation.

We all need to eat more vegetables, which are natural detoxifying agents. The best vegetables for your bowel are squash—zucchini, yellow crook-neck, and summer squash. Baked banana squash is a favorite in Europe, and it is wonderfully soothing to the bowel. All yellow fruits and vegetables tend to be laxative. All green leafy vegetables, rich in chlorophyll and iron, are cleansing to the bowel.

The Grape Diet, on page 33, is a good detoxifying diet. If you are holding down an eight-hour, regular job, you can use my Eleven-Day Elimination Regimen or my Grape Diet while you continue to work, exercise, and take hikes and walks, but it is best to rest as much as possible.

FASTING

Fasting is the quickest way of bringing about elimination in the body and the fastest way of getting toxic materials out of the body. This is done through complete rest . . . physical, mental, and spiritual.

As we let the body rest, it develops tone and vitality, more than is possible by any other procedure. Rest gives us the vitality we need to throw off toxic material and to eliminate the debris that has been accumulated over a period of years. We can literally get rid of toxic accumulations through a fast. We find that there are many ways to fast. I think the better way is to take a half glass of water every hour and a half throughout the day. If it is a hot day, you may need more water, and it is all right since you perspire more. Be sure not to take big gulps of water at one time. The water should be cool and not ice cold.

Take daily warm water enemas the first few days, then reduce this to every other day or every third or fourth day, depending on the length of time you fast. While you are fasting, you should rest as much as possible. If you hike or walk, do it on level ground. Do nothing to the point of tiring. This is important in fasting.

Breaking a Fast

The best way to break a fast is to go one or two days on juices, either vegetable or fruit, for every five to seven days on water. Take one 8-ounce glass of juice every three hours. You should have stopped using the enemas one or two days before breaking the fast. One of your most important goals now is to work toward regular, healthy, bowel movements.

After two days of juices, start the first thing in the morning of the third day with sliced or peeled oranges. The bulk of an orange is one of the finest things for the bowel. If you do not want to use oranges, you can use a finely shredded carrot that has been steamed until it is wilted—steamed just one minute or a minute and a half to just wilt it. This helps clean out toxic materials. You can have oranges for breakfast and steamed carrots for lunch. Then, for the evening meal, you can enjoy a small salad.

The next day you can have fresh fruit (citrus or any other fruit) for breakfast along with juice. Have juice as a 10:00 A.M. snack. For lunch you should have a small garden salad and juice. Have another glass of juice at 3:00 P.M. At the evening meal, you can have a salad, one cooked vegetable, and a glass of juice.

The next day continue with the same regimen, except that you may have an extra vegetable at lunch and again at supper if desired.

The first day you start on Dr. Jensen's Regular Diet, leave out the starches, but include them thereafter.

If you go on a fourteen-day water fast, it would be well for you to consider going three days on juices before starting on foods again.

If you are taking enemas during your fast, make sure you stop three or four days before you start eating solid foods. Then begin working toward natural bowel movements again.

And remember . . . no supplements on the fasting program. Vitamins and minerals are not assimilated when taken without food.

One Day a Week Fast

If you decide to follow a one day a week fast, you can use juices or fruit instead of water only. Many people like to fast one day a week. This is perfectly all right if you rest that day . . . but you MUST rest! You cannot expect to get the good yielded by a fast if you use all your energy in activities. Don't leave yourself depleted of energy by working on a day that you elect to fast.

HIGH-FIBER SUPPLEMENTS

Most diets can include high-fiber foods and supplements. There are commercial bulks in the market, for example, Today's Health, Citrucel, and many brands of powdered or ground psyllium seeds. All of these can be purchased in health food stores. Follow directions. You may find that to begin with you will have to use laxative foods to help move the high-fiber supplement along. Or it may be desirable to take flaxseed tea enemas (see page 35).

Sonne #7 is Bentonite, a very effective detoxifying liquid clay, and Sonne #9 is simply a bulk. When used with the eleven-day elimination diet, these products assist in producing the most thorough elimination possible.

We must watch for impactions in the bowel and sometimes bulk furthers these impactions. A lazy bowel many times does not move bulk along very well. It may need massage and enemas to help move it.

There are many different kinds of diets and it might be well to realize that just taking a fruit breakfast every day will help you to improve regularity and detoxify the body. My Health and Harmony Food regimen is half eliminating (detoxifying) and half building.

Extra juices in the diet will also help elimination. The juices can be taken at ten in the morning and at three in the afternoon.

Your ultimate goal must be to get off diets. . . . It is very important to realize that the diets I am recommending are temporary diets that help eliminate toxic material. There are many people on diets all the time and eliminating all the time. This leads to vitamin and mineral deficiencies. Some people never have enough building foods going into the body so that damaged tissues are not being replaced. This is not a balanced way of eating. This is why I have included in this book my descriptions of a healthy way of living. You must get OFF diets and on to a healthy way of living. That is not only for foods but for exercise and other lifestyle factors too.

Working to produce a healing crisis in the body is very important. However, you don't have to do it immediately. When a person comes under my care, I work for a healing crisis as soon as possible, considering the patient's level of health, activities, job, and consciousness. You can develop a healing crisis by following a healthy way to live and giving up all habits that interfere with good health. When you give up junk foods and a junk lifestyle and come into a right way of life, your body automatically molds into what you eat and how you live. So a healing crisis will develop of its own accord. The reversal process has already started the moment you begin to use the herb teas and add more fruits and vegetables to your diet.

MASTER CHLOROPHYLL ELIMINATION REGIMEN

This is a regimen of just plain water, preferably distilled water, adding one teaspoon of liquid chlorophyll to each glass of water and drinking it every three hours. This is a cleansing diet where we are adding iron (always found in nature with chlorophyll) and gathering all the oxygen we are breathing so that we can burn up toxic waste. Oxygen is carried to cells by iron as found in the blood. Liquid chlorophyll is usually extracted from alfalfa leaves, which is one of the highest vegetable sources of iron, which picks up oxygen from the lungs. Doing this for three or four days is a wonderful prefasting or predieting procedure. I consider this to be the master cleansing diet for all catarrhal conditions. We find that catarrh is most effectively eliminated from the body in the presence of greens.

REDUCING DIETS

There are some reducing diets that we would like to include here for both vegetarians and meat-eaters. Those who go on the meat-eater's reducing diet will lose more weight and take it off faster than those who use the vegetarian diet. We have used both diets for some years, and they really do take the weight off.

I usually recommend going one week on the reducing diet, then one week on the regular diet, alternating for a period of two months. This way we can lose weight on the reducing diet and support our health by balancing out the regular diet.

There are strict reducing diets following regular reducing diets if you would like to lose in a hurry and would like to get off more weight as you go along.

Reducing Diet for Meat Users

Alternate this diet with Dr. Jensen's Health and Harmony Food Regimen for eight weeks (two months).

You may use lamb, fish, lean beef, or poultry. Avoid fatty meats. Bake, broil, or roast fish, poultry, and meat. The fish should be a white fish (one that has fins and scales).

Always use sliced ripe tomato or grapefruit sections when you eat meat, poultry, or fish. Use canned tomatoes only when you can't get the fresh ones.

If you do not like meat, use other proteins such as eggs, cottage cheese, gelatin mold, skim milk, soy milk, tofu, low-fat yogurt, and rice milk.

All vegetables should be from the 5 Percent Carbohydrate Vegetables chart outlined on page 29.

Drink in between meals, *only*. This should be one hour before or two hours after meals. Use KB-11 or Cleaver tea (2 cups daily).

The suggested eating plan for a week includes:

Breakfast: One fresh fruit and one or two eggs or cottage cheese.

5 PERCENT CARBOHYDRATE VEGETABLES			
Artichokes	Cucumber	Radishes	String beans
Asparagus	Dandelion	Rhubarb	Swiss chard
Beet greens	Eggplant	Sauerkraut	Tomatoes
Broccoli	Endive	(not	Turnip
Brussels	Escarole	canned)	greens
sprouts	Leeks	Sea kale	Vegetable
Cabbage	Lettuce	Sorrel	marrow
Cauliflower	Mushroom	Spinach	Watercress
Celery	Mustard	Sprouts	
Chard	greens	(alfalfa,	
Chicory	Okra	mung, etc.)	

Lunch: Brown rice, one vegetable, and salad.

Dinner: Meat or fish with tomato or grapefruit, and one vegetable (if desired).

Other meal suggestions include:

1. One cup low-fat milk, 1 tablespoon sesame seed meal, ⅓ avocado, and one fruit. Blend.
2. One cup low-fat milk, watercress or romaine lettuce (liquefy); salad; fish and tomato.
3. One cup low-fat milk, watercress or romaine lettuce (liquefy); salad; fish and tomato.
4. Fruit and cheese.
5. Apples and cottage cheese.

You may use rice cakes or Ry-Krisp once in a while.

Strict Reducing Diet for Meat Users

Use only this menu:

Breakfast: One fresh fruit and one or two eggs.

Lunch: Vegetable and salad.

Dinner: Meat or fish with tomato or grapefruit.

Reducing Diet for Vegetarians

Alternate this diet with Dr. Jensen's Health and Harmony Food Regimen every other week for eight weeks (two months).

Drink in between meals only. This should be at least one hour before or two hours after meals. Use KB-11 or Cleaver tea (two cups daily).

Always use sliced ripe tomato or grapefruit sections with proteins at dinner. Use canned tomatoes only when you can't get the fresh ones.

Use proteins such as eggs, cottage cheese, gelatin, soy tofu, and low-fat yogurt.

All vegetables should be from the 5 Percent Carbohydrate Vegetable chart on page 29.

Suggested eating plan for a week:

Breakfast: One fresh fruit and one or two eggs or cottage cheese.

Lunch: Brown rice and one vegetable and salad.

Dinner: Protein with tomato or grapefruit and one vegetable, if desired.

Other meal suggestions include:

1. One cup soy milk or low-fat milk, 1 tablespoon sesame seed meal, ⅓ avocado, and one fruit. Liquefy.
2. Fruit and cheese.
3. Apple and low-fat yogurt.
4. One cup low-fat milk, watercress or romaine lettuce (liquefy); salad with cottage cheese and tomato (or use four to six watercress tablets per meal).

You may use rice cakes or Ry-Krisp once in a while, and chlorella tablets will help balance every meal.

Strict Reducing Diet for Vegetarians

Use only this menu:

Breakfast: One fresh fruit and one or two eggs.

Lunch: Vegetable salad.

Dinner: Soy protein with tomato or grapefruit.

☯ Warning

In my opinion, it is very difficult to retrace and do a good job in tubercular cases. While these cases have usually gone through a suppression, I think it is well not to awaken it again and bring it to the elimination stage. However, a person can go on to fairly good health by living a sensible life and by keeping away from the extremes as we take many people through the elimination diets. Also, anyone with diabetes or hypoglycemia should diet only under supervision by their doctor.

CARROT JUICE DIET

Let me inform you that taking carrot juice only constitutes a diet. The time comes when you must get off it because it will not sustain life adequately. It is not a perfect food. It is not well balanced, nor does it have all the minerals, vitamins, lipids, and proteins necessary for building a completely new body. Tissue that needs protein will not get enough of it from the carrots.

I don't think there's any particular juice that will cure anything . . . but I believe the rest you give your body allows it the opportunity to reverse the disease and recover your health. It's the rest from food and the simple diet that does the trick. The lack of too many food mixtures and less demand made on our digestive and elimination system helps us to overcome disease.

Some people go on the carrot juice diet for a week, some for two weeks, and some can go a month without any trouble. As is often the case, it is best to go on these diets under the supervision and guidance of a doctor or your physician.

Most carrot juice diets involve taking one glass of carrot juice every three hours (or more if you like). You can do this for ten days, twenty days, or even longer. I had one man on carrot juice for a full year. That is a long time! This particular man had cancer of the bowel, but through the carrot juice diet he got rid of it.

Dr. H. E. Kirshner, who wrote the book *Live Food Juices* (H. E. Kirschner Publications, Monrovia, Calif., 1975) came to my office to talk over this man's case because he found out that I had kept him on juices for a long time. The man passed off mucus and catarrh continually from that bowel. It was almost unbelievable what was eliminated. This was simply accumulated toxic material that was necessary for him to get rid of.

Sometimes enemas can be used with this diet.

GRAPE DIET

Four pounds of grapes a day is a good amount for a grape diet, and some of my patients have averaged a pound or so every three hours. These grapes should not be the seedless white or red grapes but the kind that have seeds since these are the most vital of all grapes. I caution my patients against using hybrid foods too much. All original fruits and vegetables were propagated by seeds. Seedless fruits are a product of crossbreeding and are not found in nature. Foods with seeds are the vital foods. So, I believe the grapes that have seeds are the best. The Concord, Fresno Beauty, red grapes, and Muscats are all good grapes to use. I don't say that you have to use the seeds. You can chew them fine if you like. A good thing to help eliminate catarrh is found in cream of tartar that surrounds grape seeds. So make sure you get all the material off the seeds when you are eating them. When chewing grape skins, you'll find that they are very bitter, but the bitterness indicates that grape skins are high in potassium. Potassium is a great cleanser in the body. Gayelord Hauser built his reputation with potassium broth. It is a great cleanser and detoxifier in the body.

I think enemas should be used, especially in the beginning of the grape diet. Toxic materials accumulate, and it is well that we keep things moving along. You can go on grapes five to ten days without any supervision, but if you stay on them longer, it is advisable to have someone around who is familiar with the grape diet. That person should be able to take care of any reaction you might have that may seem strange to you . . . many times these reactions are nothing more than a healing crisis or an elimination.

WATERMELON FLUSH

There are times during the watermelon season that we can use watermelon as a good elimination diet food. Going on watermelon for three, four, or five days can be a wonderful diuretic. We find that it helps to take out a lot of the debris in the colon, and the extra water picks up toxic materials and carries them off.

POTATO PEEL BROTH

Potato peel broth is a high potassium broth and is one of the best broths I know for taking care of extreme acids in the body, especially rheumatic and arthritic acids. Taking two cups a day for one month, or even two months, between meals, is tolerated by most people along with their regular diet. We find that this helps neutralize acids that have accumulated over long periods of time. It helps get rid of the toxic wastes that have settled into various parts of the body and neutralize the acids that attack the joints. We find that it is a wonderful aid in getting rid of rheumatic pains in the body. This broth should be used right along with a good, healthy way of living.

HERB TEAS

Any of the herb teas are helpful. Think of their value and try to relate them to the particular problem you have. For instance, for weak kidneys, there is no reason why you should not use shave

---

∞ My Crisis Broth

I find the thing to do in the time of a health crisis is to rely more on vegetables. Sometimes taking too much of the fruit juices forces an elimination too rapidly, too intensely, and vegetables are easier on our body's systems. I put most of my patients who go through the healing crisis on potato peel broth for one to three days. We lose potassium salts in our body through the elimination process. We replace this with potassium from potato peel broth.

---

grass tea, parsley tea, or kidney and bladder teas available from the health food stores.

A good eliminating tea for the kidneys is made from juniper berries. Mash them, pour a cup of hot water on them, let stand until the boiling water is just slightly warm, and drink the excellent tea. You may add a little honey if you wish. Using this three times in twenty-four hours makes a wonderful kidney detoxifier. You can also cook some fresh asparagus in water and take a half teacup of the water three times a day.

Peppermint tea is good for stomach trouble as is chamomile tea.

If you have lung catarrh, comfrey tea and fenugreek tea may be used two or three times daily.

Flaxseed tea is one of the great elimination and healing teas for the bowel. It is useful for inflammation or irritations of the bowel, as well as for stomach ulcers.

Steep one teaspoon of flaxseed in a cup of hot water and let stand until it becomes somewhat "mucilaginous." In some cases, it is desirable to drink the liquid and discard the seeds.

Flaxseed tea is of good use in enemas. Some people find that taking plain water enemas is irritating to the bowel, but by using a combination of one pint flaxseed tea and one teaspoon liquid chlorophyll, they are able to get good results without disturbance or pain. This can be used daily as needed.

There are other detoxifying diets too. One, for instance, is cleansing the gallbladder with beet juice or beet juice plus a little olive oil.

Remember, one of our goals is to get to the place where we use everything possible to build the strength and resistance of tissues so that they will eliminate toxic substances.

When I mention that it is not well to be on an alkalinizing diet continually and that we may produce an overalkalinization through these diets, I recognize that this can be helpful in dealing with an abnormal condition in the body. Proteins and starches added to the diet keep us from becoming overalkalinized. The urine is supposed to be acid. If it has become alkaline, it can often be a sign that we are living on too many fruits and vegetables. While Dr. D. C. Jarvis, author of *Folk Medicine* (Fawcett Book Group, 1970), used a tablespoon of apple cider vinegar in a glass of water to bring the urine back to normal, we believe the greatest correction comes when we change our diet and lifestyle.

KNEIPP LEG BATHS

Go outside where you can stand on grass or sand. Take a water hose, without spray attachment, and starting from the toes go up the right leg to the groin, then around to the back of the right leg and down to the heel. Repeat on the left leg from toes to groin, around to the back of the thigh and down the left leg to the heel. Do each leg only one time up and down and do only one time each day. Do not dry with a towel. Walk on sand or grass until the legs and feet are dry, approximately ten minutes. Drying with a towel would negate the beneficial effect.

As soon as you start the detoxification process and begin putting your mind in good order, you will realize that you are on your way to building a better body. I know it's impossible to live the perfect life. But you'll find as you face life with a more enlightened attitude, determined to live in harmony with nature, many aspects of your life and health will be lifted up.

EXERCISE

I have used every way possible to improve elimination for my patients. For example, I teach them that exercise develops tone in tissues, and strong tissues eliminate better. So, nutrition and exercise help each other.

Playful recreation is good, and when I speak of this, I mean water exercises, baseball, handball, hiking, and basketball, to name just a few. They detoxify the body. Exercise induces sweating and promotes circulation of blood and lymph throughout the tissues. It quickens the elimination of toxic waste and rebuilding of cell structure. There are bed exercises that you may have to get acquainted with if you cannot get out and run, jump, or jog. There are exercises that can be used under all conditions . . . in open air, in water, and even in a bed or wheelchair. I'm referring to exercises such as isometrics. You have to be almost completely ossified not to be able to exercise.

Isometric exercises involving tension and relaxation, pushing and pulling, can be very effective in detoxification. There are exercises to help the lymph glands around the neck. There are midsection exercises for the bowels.

There are liver exercises involving twisting, bending down, and turning the body from side to side. Slant board exercises are excellent, in which we bring the legs up to the chest, squeezing the abdominal muscles. Try bicycling your legs upside down in bed or on the slant board. Detoxification also improves under the influence of sunshine. You could have a helio gym, so to speak, where you can do exercises in sunshine, in the nude if possible.

Jumping and rope skipping are wonderful in helping to detoxify the body. You should also investigate jogging and running machines like those in fitness centers. This is a great instrument to use if you can't get outside to run or walk.

Rowing a boat is wonderful for the lungs and the chest. Bicycling is wonderful for the legs. Consider horseback riding. These exercises help the stomach, bowel, liver, and the circulation. And, of course, consider the social side of your nature.

We are constantly developing a health spa around us by building an effective detoxifying program. A certain amount of sleep is necessary for good detoxification. Try getting to bed early a few nights. I've seen people with swollen ankles that wouldn't respond much to treatments, but going to bed early and lying prone helped greatly.

FOUR ELIMINATION CHANNELS

Bowel Toning

It is necessary to have clean, iron-rich blood for the repair and rebuilding of good tissue, but this tissue must also have tone. I believe that food alone is not the cure-all that we need in the reversal process. By reversal process, I mean the reversal of disease until it is gone. I advise different exercises, especially for the bowel and the abdominal organs, to build up the tone so that they may function better. A tired, flabby bowel cannot eliminate well. Therefore, I teach my patients to build up the tone through corrective exercises. The exercises that are best for the abdominal tract are as follows:

The Chest Leg Pull Up Exercise. This involves sitting on the edge of a chair with your shoulders almost touching the back of the chair and the heels almost touching the floor while your hands grasp the side of the chair. Lift the knees to the chest, straighten out the legs but do not touch the floor, and bring the legs up and back at least two or three times (and up to ten to fifteen times as you grow stronger).

The Alley Cat Exercise. This is another good toning exercise. While standing, lift one leg, bend the knee, and bring it up and over in front of the abdomen and other leg. Alternate with the other leg and do this exercise ten to fifteen times.

The Rubber Ball Exercise. This is a wonderful exercise to do while lying in bed. Using a ball, like a tennis ball or handball, roll it around the abdomen twenty-five times beginning on the right side and going completely around in a circle over the abdomen. Press the ball as you roll it, and tense the abdominal muscles in response.

Slant Board Exercises. These will help all lazy bowels, even those with diverticulosis. It's a great help in prolapsus and colon stasis, relieving gas pressure and stimulating the vital nerve centers of the brain. I do not advise using the slant board when there is high blood pressure, heart disease, internal bleeding, hemorrhages, or wherever exercises of any kind are contraindicated for any abdominal problem.

When there is a lack of tone in the abdominal muscles (abs), we can expect prolapsus of the abdominal organs. The heart, lacking tone, cannot pump blood properly throughout the body, and blood does not have sufficient pressure to work uphill against gravity to reach the brain tissues.

There are people who apparently have tried everything to get well and all their organs are still working under par. Many people do not realize that the quickening force for every organ of the body comes from the brain. People whose occupations require them to sit or stand continually are unable to get the blood into the brain tissues because a flaccid, underexercised heart cannot force the blood uphill. If we deny the brain tissues the blood it needs, in time every organ in our body will suffer.

The heart gets its innervation and control from the brain and continues its rhythmic pumping because of it. No organ can function without the brain. I attribute the success of my healing work to the very fact that I recognize that the brain must be fed properly. Slant board exercises are absolutely necessary to regain perfect health.

There are many cases where the slant board is contraindicated. It is best to seek professional advice before starting too strenuous a program. If you haven't done much exercising of the abdominal muscles, it is well to take these exercises slowly, and gradually increase them as you get stronger.

Do not use the board in cases of high blood pressure, cancer in the pelvic cavity, appendicitis, ulcers of the stomach or intestines, or pregnancy, unless under the care of a physician.

The slant board exercises are practically the same as other lying-down exercises. The most important exercise is to hold on to the sides of the board, bringing the knees up to the chest. This forces all the abdominal organs up toward the shoulders.

While in this position, twist the head from side to side and in all directions, thus utilizing the extra force to circulate blood to all areas of the brain and head. Drawing the knees to the chest on a slant board brings the stomach and abdominal organs up toward the chest, which strengthens and tones them.

Slant board exercises are especially good in cases of inflammations and congestions above the shoulders, such as sinus trouble,

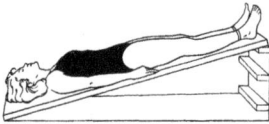

1. Lie flat on your back, allowing gravity to help shift abdominal organs into their proper positions and letting blood circulate to the head. Lie on board at least 10 minutes. This basic position should begin and end all series of exercises.

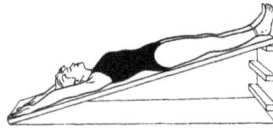

2. While lying on your back, stretch the abdomen by raising arms above head. Next, lower arms to sides. Raise and lower arms 10 to 15 times. This stretches the abdominal muscles and pulls the abdomen down toward the shoulders.

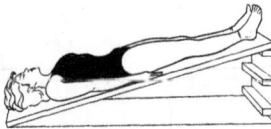

3. *If you are in great shape and under age forty, you may be able to proceed safely with the following exercise. Otherwise, wait until you have exercised for at least two weeks, then proceed carefully, taking care to avoid excessive abdominal strain. Consult your doctor if you are uncertain.* Take a deep breath and hold it. Still holding your breath, alternately flex (contract) and relax abdominal muscles 5 times. You should feel your abdomen pressing upward toward your shoulders as you flex and feel it dropping down a little as you relax. Take a normal breath, then repeat the exercise 10 to 15 times, breathing normally between sets.

Continued

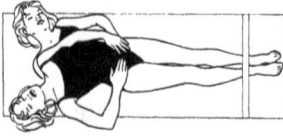

4. Pat abdomen vigorously with open hands. Lean to one side and then to the other, patting 10 to 15 times on each side. Reverse sides 3 or 4 times. Next, bring the body to a sitting position, using the abdominal muscles. Return to lying position.

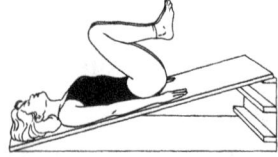

5. Holding onto the board, bring knees up toward chest. While in this position, (a) turn head from side to side 5 or 6 times, then (b) lift head slightly and rotate in circles 3 or 4 times. Reverse rotation. Repeat each set 2 or 3 times.

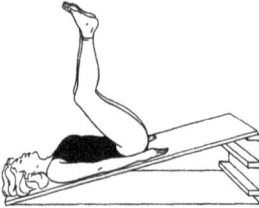

6. Holding onto the board, lift legs to a vertical position. Rotate legs outward in opposite circles 8 to 10 times. Change directions, rotating circles inward. Increase to 25 times after a week or two of exercising.

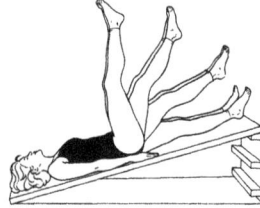

7. Raise legs to a vertical position. Keeping knees straight, slowly lower left leg to the board, then right leg. Raise each leg then lower each leg 15 to 25 times. Next, with legs in a vertical position, slowly lower both together to the board. Repeat 3 or 4 times.

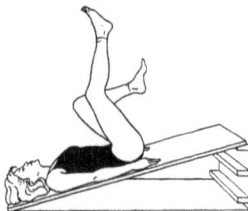

8. Raise legs to a vertical position. Bicycle legs in air 15 to 25 times. Do this at a slow pace at first, increasing speed gradually through the first week or two of regular exercise.

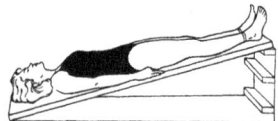

9. Lying flat on your back, relax completely, letting the blood circulate. Hold this position 5 to 15 minutes.

vision and eye problems, head eczema, ear conditions, and similar troubles. Slant board exercises are beneficial to those who may have poor blood circulation, fatigue, dizziness, failing memory, and paralysis. Most people can easily tolerate a slant angle in which the foot end of the board is at chair height for all exercises. If dizziness occurs, the foot end of the board could be lowered to a more comfortable height. Exercise only five minutes a day to begin with. Gradually increase time spent on board to ten minutes. You may find it convenient to exercise on the slant board ten minutes at three o'clock in the afternoon and again just before going to bed. In bed, lift the buttocks up a little to allow the organs to return to a normal position.

Skin Brushing (Dry)

The elimination organs should always be taken care of first in working toward better health. Skin brushing is most important to get the skin to eliminate properly. I believe skin brushing is one of the finest of all "baths." No soap can wash the skin as clean as the new skin you have under the old. You make new skin constantly, your whole life long. The skin will be as clean as is the blood that nourishes it.

Skin brushing removes this top layer of skin. This helps to eliminate uric acid crystals, catarrh, and various other acids from the body. The skin should eliminate about two pounds of waste acids daily. Keep the skin active. No one can have truly clean, healthy skin after wearing clothes most of the time unless they brush their skin.

Use a dry, long-handled vegetable-bristle, flesh-massage brush. It is not an expensive brush. *Do not use nylon.* Use this brush dry, first thing in the morning when you arise before bathing or dressing. Use it in any direction all over the whole body except the face. You can use a special, softer brush for the face.

Lung Exercising

Hiking, running, walking, swimming, bending, twisting, and all aerobic exercises help the lungs to breathe more deeply and take in more oxygen. Quick inhalations with slow exhalations help exercise the lung structure.

Kidney and Bladder Cleansing

For taking care of the kidneys, use the instructions for liquid intake (especially water) and elimination diets and procedures as brought forth in this book.

One simple daily kidney-bladder cleansing should be done every day by taking two or three glasses of liquids or water before breakfast every morning. This exercises the bladder and eliminates urine and residue that has accumulated during the night and also tones the bladder. This is especially helpful when people pass the age of fifty.

This takes care of all four elimination channels—bowel, skin, lungs, and kidneys—mechanically. Water treatments and massage, physiotherapy, and other forms of therapy may be used to hasten the development of proper tissue tone and activity in the body. Always think, however, in terms of developing the whole body rather than just one tissue or one organ.

CHAPTER 4

DETOXIFICATION

My approach to detoxification is the natural way . . .
without drugs . . . the "Nature Cure."

There is a difference between the activity of drugs and the activity of a nature cure. I am not going to say that one is better than the other, but there is a life style that appeals to each of us . . . as some people like Collies, some like Scotties, or some like to be Baptists, some like to be Catholics. There seems to be something for everyone. I feel that there is value in each search for truth and personal significance, and I feel that no matter what path you choose, the result will be for your soul growth through experiences.

While we are growing through experience, some of us realize that much of our daily lives are out of tune with nature and nature's laws. We may have a thought that we have strayed from the innocence and simplicity of the Garden of Eden. We may find out the hard way that our lifestyle and diet are not conducive to making the best body or the best health. We come to realize that we have accumulated unwanted "baggage" in our bodies, minds, and spirits that is getting in the way of our search for happiness and peace of mind.

DO YOU KNOW WHAT IT IS
TO FEEL WONDERFUL?

I don't know if many really know how great it is to feel good . . . feel wonderful . . . and, most of all, feel healthy. I believe that health is not everything, but without health everything else is nothing! Without good health, you cannot spend your money and enjoy it. Without good health, you cannot have a fulfilling marriage or bring up children properly. You have to recognize that there is a price to be paid when you follow the path that leads to "feeling wonderful." It is not an easy one, but the results from cooperating with nature are always forthcoming and are usually long lasting.

According to my nature cure approach to health and healing, if we suppress natural elimination processes, driving toxic material into the body or causing it to be retained, eventually chronic disease will develop. What we need to do is to reverse the disease and accumulation of toxic materials in the body. You can only do this by detoxifying the body . . . giving it a rest, taking in more liquids, and draining off the catarrh, toxic materials, and accumulations that are found in the body by bringing them to the "running stage." The word *catarrh* is derived from Greek words meaning "to flow down." When you bring dried catarrh back to a lightly flowing stage, your body begins to cleanse itself. Healing leads to cleansing and cleansing leads to healing.

In contrast to nature cure, drugs are man-made chemical compositions that have specific effects on the body, some good and some bad. All doctors and drug manufacturers will tell you that drugs have undesirable side effects. Many drugs suppress the body's natural eliminations and mask symptoms of disease.

Adding iron to the diet helps to eliminate drug residues in the body that hinder natural healing processes. Iron in the blood attracts oxygen from the air inhaled into the lungs. We find that iron is most necessary to draw enough oxygen out of the air to increase the body's energy level and boost the metabolism until organs, glands, and tissues are able to throw off these toxic materials in the body. Iron is found in blackberries, raspberries, loganberries, and all greens as well as in meat, poultry, and fish.

Our goal in nature cure is to liquefy and drain off toxic deposits from the various tissues of the body and move these toxic materials to the eliminative organs. Withdrawal from certain drugs may bring on symptoms and elimination processes that are very severe. They may be almost intolerable. But in order to get well, some people will have to go through with it.

Many people under detoxification have cut out their coffee and developed a caffeine withdrawal headache. We have to get rid of all the caffeine, nicotine, drug residues, heavy metals, and other toxins that have accumulated in the tissues. We may have to go through the coffee headaches to get well. We may have to go through alcohol withdrawal. The same applies to all the drugs or anything else that has settled in the body and interferes with health and healing.

People say that nature cure takes a long time. Yes, it does, but a chronic disease takes a long time to develop, too. We have to understand that the body works according to natural law, and, in the reversal process, as the body cleanses itself we find that we go back over the same course that the disease followed as it developed. This conforms to Hering's Law of Cure: "All cure is from the head down, from the inside out, and in reverse order as the symptoms first appeared."

To take care of asthma in the reversal process, the patient always goes through symptoms of hay fever and the flu again . . . tiredness, aching bones, fever. The symptoms all come back briefly, but if the patient goes through with this process, they get a healthy, well body.

Suffering does not always come only physically . . . it can come mentally and spiritually. I feel very depressed when I see a child with asthma being given an all-day sucker or an ice-cream cone. Sweets are among the very things that produce the trouble! The big problem here is ignorance. When you know better, isn't it sad to see a thing like this happen? Some people just don't know any better. So they have to learn in the school of hard knocks and through terrible experiences.

I often find that the average person who gets sick of being sick turns to the natural methods and to nature cure.

Many people just want to get rid of their present symptoms, and we find that as soon as they get rid of them, they go back on the same wrong living habits, then feel or believe they are happy.

When you come with me, you have to clean up your life! You clean up your mind, you clean up your ideals, straighten out your direction in life, and strive for a new body. All this involves healing crises and elimination processes. There are many people who come to me with a coated tongue, which is a sign that they are loaded to the gills, so to speak, with toxic materials. It means the liver is toxic and the bowel is not eliminating properly. The lungs are loaded with catarrh, mucus, and phlegm. To eliminate this material, we have to start the process of detoxification.

How long does detoxification take? I think it is best to consider doing it for two or three weeks on whatever program you want to go on, then adopt a healthy way of living. Eventually, you should come back to another detoxifying program according to the amount of weight you gained, the condition of your body, if you can stand it again, and so forth.

Don't try to do the whole thing at one time! It is best to do these programs under a doctor's care.

A man came in one day complaining that he had bad breath, his vision was becoming poor, he was hard of hearing, and his tongue was coated as he had never seen it before. He said it had all happened in the past four or five months. I asked him about his bowel, and he said in the last four or five months the bowel hadn't moved well and elimination had practically stopped. He had to resort to enemas and laxatives, and he now wondered what was wrong. He noticed that the odor from his body had become very strong, and that his wife had started to complain about it. It was time for a detoxification program, so I started him out by going through the Eleven-Day Elimination Regimen. This might not fit everybody. You must be wise in your selection.

You can go on carrot juice for five days, or take the grape diet for ten or twelve days as outlined in chapter 3. You can go on a short fast, or you can go on a long fast if you are capable and have had experience in fasting. However, I do not think anyone should go on a long water fast by themselves. Always follow your doctor's advice in that regard.

Allergies are helped through the detoxification program. We find that all cases involving catarrhal discharges are helped by an elimination diet program. This kind of program is the first thing to think about for any discharge or pain in the body. Go on as little food as possible and undertake a detoxification program.

Sometimes when we want to eliminate and detoxify, it is well to leave the environment in which the health problems developed. It is best to be with happy people and develop a new attitude toward life. This means that you have to get away from mean, irritable people and start a new life for yourself. Happiness is part of a good elimination program. People need happiness, love, peace, and harmony today more than anything else.

We should never stop a catarrh, phlegm, or mucus discharge in the body. To stop this discharge is what we call suppression. We recognize that in suppression of natural elimination we are traveling on to a more chronic disease. We give the body its will to cleanse and purify itself and never stop a discharge. To use a treatment, food, drug, or lifestyle habit that stops the discharge is to suppress the symptoms or disease.

Detoxifying programs are helpful in nearly every disease. They are indicated in practically all lung problems. Some diseases require special precautions, for example, tuberculosis, diabetes, and epilepsy.

Convulsions can develop very fast under an elimination program, and we should make sure someone who knows how to handle them is in attendance. Convulsions are involuntary muscle contractions. There are numerous possible causes, and the release of toxins during a fast or elimination diet may bring about chemical changes in the brain that disrupt brain centers and trigger convulsions. In diabetes, we find that a person could fall into a coma, and it is necessary to have them under competent supervision. Colitis responds well to a detoxifying program. Constipation (bowel stasis) is the first thing to take care of when detoxifying.

CARE OF THE BOWEL THROUGH ENEMAS AND OTHER CLEANSING METHODS

We do not detoxify the body just by eliminating bowel wastes. There is more to it than that! We have to recognize that cells must be fed and that vital energy has to be built up in the body. There has to be a detoxification going on in the liver and all other internal organs as well as in the bowel, lymph glands, lungs, kidneys, and even the skin. As the elimination channels are detoxified and cleaned up, other parts of the body begin releasing their toxins.

The first thing I would like to point out is that detoxification takes place normally in the body when we have good health. However, very few people have good health. Many people, having a fever, rely only on enemas. They don't realize that there are herb teas that act as diuretics, increasing elimination of toxic waste through the kidneys.

As we strive for good health and build structure and fiber strength in our body tissues, the body will eliminate better. We throw off the toxic wastes that have been absorbed into our inherently weak tissues when we were tired, fatigued, overworked, and low in resistance. There are many metabolic wastes we have to detoxify and eliminate. There may be acids that develop from worry, hate, and fear. Catarrhal conditions develop in the body from poor diets or when people have taken drugs. Through an elimination program, we can start what we call a withdrawal of drug deposits and other toxins in the body.

I want to emphasize that enemas, colonic cleansing, and a relatively recent process called colemas can play a very important role in body detoxification. A colema is a bowel-cleansing method intermediately between an enema and a colonic. It is more thorough than an enema but not as powerful or risky as a colonic. Bowel cleansing can seldom be adequately done in less than a week, but when it is completed, all other eliminative systems or channels become much more efficient at getting rid of toxins.

THE IMPORTANCE OF THE HEALING CRISIS

When this elimination process is developed and toxic materials are ready to be thrown off by a strong body, we have literally earned a healing crisis. That healing crisis is what we need for nature's version of what we call a "cure."

> *Give me a healing crisis and I will cure any disease.*
> —Dr. Henry Lindlahr
>
> *Give me a fever and I will cure any disease.*
> —Hippocrates, the Father of Medicine

It is during these healing crises that we develop fevers. When we first experience these crises, they seem to be disease crises. They actually manifest the same symptoms. However, onset of the healing crisis usually develops while the patient feels terrific, while a disease crisis develops after a period of poor health. We find that a healing crisis brings on more elimination through all five of the eliminating organs (skin, bowel, lungs, lymph, and kidneys) than it does in a disease crisis. The bowels invariably work all too perfectly in a healing crisis, but this does not happen in a disease crisis. That is why enemas are given when you are sick. However, you don't need to think about enemas in a healing crisis because usually the bowel works very well.

For a healing crisis to happen, the cells have to be fed and internal organs have to develop integrity of tissue so that they can throw off toxic encumbrances through the strong exertion of every organ, gland, and tissue of the body.

There is one thing you should remember about the diets I have been recommending: Eventually you will have to get off diets. Most of them are for detoxification purposes, for elimination, for weight reduction, or for chemically rebalancing the body. The time comes when you just have to move on to a healthy way of living and eating, leaving diets and all other temporary health-boosting procedures behind.

A little thing to consider here is that elimination may go too fast for some people. They may lose weight too rapidly and become weak on the diet or other cleansing procedure. We find that sometimes taking too much fruit and fruit juice (especially citrus) on the diet will produce this condition. Remember that vegetables carry off acids and act on the body much slower than do fruits. Fruits stir up the acids, and many times we have to be careful about taking too much fruit juice. We find that citrus fruit is high in its life-giving energies and can stir up toxic materials very quickly. If our elimination channels are not prepared to take out the stirred-up acids that the citrus causes in the body, we may experience cramps, pain, and fevers from placing too much stress on organs of elimination.

There are four starches that produce the least amount of catarrh when used in one's diet, and as part of our cleansing strategy, I think we have to consider giving up wheat and oatmeal. I am convinced that it is the gluten in these two products that produce much of the heavy catarrhal conditions in the body. Wheat, by the way, puts on fat. So does oatmeal. And we find that the four starches that I am going to recommend will not put on weight and will not produce catarrh. They are rye, rice, yellow cornmeal, and millet. All four of these are wonderfully nourishing whole cereal grains.

∽ Remember this . . .

A long fast should be under the supervision of a doctor. Detoxification is like tearing down the walls of an old building. There comes a time when you have to rebuild, and that results from a new eating regimen. Eventually you have to get off the diet idea and go on to a healthy way of living. It is best to go from the elimination diet to a healthy way of living, then another month or so on an elimination diet, and then back to a healthy way of living.

One man told me he had been on a grapefruit diet and found that it helped his sinuses tremendously. Then he said, "I heard you give the carrot juice diet here." I said, "Yes, we can give you carrot juice as a diet." He said, "I would like to go three weeks on carrot juice." So he went three weeks on carrot juice, then found out that watermelon is very high in silicon and is supposed to be very good for catarrh problems. So he went three weeks on a watermelon diet. When he was finished with that, the grape season came in and, of course, grapes are so good in catarrh problems, he went on a three-week grape diet. This is too much. Don't spend your life chasing diets.

You cannot build the body on a detoxifying diet, an elimination diet, or through fasting. You must find a way of maintaining good health through proper living and balanced eating. Diets come from doctors and hospitals to apply remedial therapy for people who are not taking good care of themselves. It is not a healthy way of living. Can you understand that?

The best food program for everyone is my Health and Harmony Food Regimen. You should learn this healthy way of living and use it at home.

PHYSICAL CHANGE CREATES A MENTAL CHANGE

A sick person is seldom happy but a well person often is! As we eliminate toxic material from the body, there is a mind change as well as a body change because we relieve the mind and brain of the stressful poison of toxic materials. We think more clearly and we're able to make decisions better. We're able to enjoy our surroundings and we see beauty as we have never seen it before.

Happiness and beauty cannot be expressed in a sick, toxic body. Sick people go around moping and say they don't feel good, nothing seems to be right, and they are irritable. I believe there are mental conditions in people that, in reality, are nothing more than toxic disturbances that interfere with proper brain and nerve activity. We have to have unimpaired nerve supply to every organ in the body. This is the number one function that must be taken care of before our body and mind can be well. The moment we supply the nerve structure with good nourishment or start eliminating toxic material that has accumulated in the body, we start feeling better and the mind functions better and clearer. When the mind works better, we find that all nerve activity works better. Everything in the body works better.

What we invariably hear from a person who undertakes detoxification is, "I am feeling better!" The feelings are cleared up in the nervous structure. Our cell structure becomes hungry, thirsty, cold, and painful at times. To clean up these conditions, we have to go through a detoxifying program to relieve cells of this debris in the body.

> *The mind cannot be set apart as an entirely disassociated entity. No mind ever existed that was entirely free from the influences of bodily processes, animal impulses, savage traditions, infantile impressions, conventional reactions, and traditional knowledge.*
>
> —Anonymous

We need outside help in our detoxifying program. We need to remove some obstacles to better health, which in our case may be coffee and doughnuts or toxins from fried foods, chemical additives from processed foods, or poisons from cigarettes or chewing tobacco. We eventually find that these things make up the debris that trap us in unhealthy lives. One of these days we will wonder just how we got so stuck in poor health and unhappiness.

If your eyes are bad, maybe they are compromised with toxins. If you cannot hear well, your inner ear probably is influenced by toxic materials from junk foods you have consumed. It is possible that every cell and every organ in your body needs rejuvenation. New blood cells are made every 120 days. You make new tissue from clean blood for a vital way of life. I also want to mention that as we eliminate the toxic materials from one organ in the body, every other organ is affected. This is because it is done through the blood. The blood contacts every cell in the body. Every organ in your body is fed and cleansed by the blood. So we must cleanse the blood. We must give our blood the right nutrients through proper diet measures.

The liver is definitely one of the first organs we should take care of. This is the organ that detoxifies and eliminates wastes more than any other organ in the body except the bowel. It does it naturally for us, but we still need to avoid foods that the liver has to detoxify, and use foods that nourish and strengthen it. Try using good natural foods in your everyday diet. Soon you will find that the liver will start to improve and detoxify more efficiently. Some foods you can eat to help the liver are cherry juice, alfalfa tablets, alfalfa tea, alfalfa greens, and chlorophyll, which is one of the greatest cleansers we have. We find that dwarf nettle broth, peppermint, and bitter greens help the liver. Dandelion greens and dandelion tea are also great cleansers for the liver.

We need to have antiseptic foods, such as white or green grapes, lemons, onions, and garlic. In addition, pineapple juice, mulberries, prickly pears, and oat straw broth are great catarrhal eliminators. We also find that silicon foods and foods high in sodium are antiseptic and acid-reducing.

The most beneficial foods for eliminating catarrh and for developing a greater quickening response of the tissues in order to throw off toxic material are to be found in our iodine foods, such as Nova Scotia dulse, carrageen, kelp, and food crops grown within fifty miles of the oceans. We find that raw goat milk is one of the foods highest in fluorine, which is especially good in reducing lung troubles and expelling lung catarrh. Fluorine is the decay-resistant element in teeth and bones and is helpful in fighting off infections. Chlorine, the cleansing element, helps eliminate pus and catarrhal conditions in the body. It is abundant in all vegetables and fruits, found everywhere sodium and potassium are present. Silicon is useful to expel pleural catarrh (the pleura is the membrane surrounding the lung). Silicon is stored in the human skin and helps keep this elimination organ active. Sodium foods are good for pus elimination also. The best sodium foods are olives, whey of any kind, okra, and celery. These are all very high in sodium, as are sun-ripened fruits and sweet fruits.

When we want to get rid of catarrh, we may use poultices and packs. Comfrey packs on infected sores are wonderful. We find that aloe vera can be used as a pack. Also, onion poultices on the neck, chest, and thyroid gland are wonderful for ridding the body of catarrhal conditions due to colds. Strong sunlight is very helpful in diminishing catarrhal conditions. Altitude, dry air, and noncatarrhal foods must also be considered. Bone set or comfrey tea is especially good in relieving flu misery and flu catarrh.

To relieve the body cells of the debris they have accumulated over a period of years through devitalized catarrh-forming foods, such as refined flour, white sugar, and products made of them, we have to start an elimination program directly involving the elimination organs.

The first and most important thing to do is to take care of the toxic material in the bowel. We must have at least 25 to 30 grams of fiber in our diet every day. We can get this from vegetable salads, fruits, and whole grains. Many people don't think that salads are necessary. Many people think that parsley is meant to be used just to decorate a plate. It was made to eat! Very few people think of steaming and eating beet greens. Spinach can be used raw or cooked. When we want to eliminate toxic materials in the body, we should eat more raw foods. I don't mean that you should get 100 percent of your foods raw, but we should eat a lot of them. Raw vegetable juices are especially good for the bowel and the liver.

Raw shredded beet is one of the best eliminators we have, and it stimulates the flow of bile from the liver and gallbladder into the intestinal tract. The greatest fiber sources are alfalfa tablets and oat bran.

Many times I recommend a pancreatic substance along with the diet to help our foods digest, and we could also use herbal digestants. I take a couple of these each meal.

Digestion is helped by adding pancreatic substance to each meal. Papaya tablets are also very good, and, they are very mild. We find that ginger can also be used. In addition, mint tea is a wonderful gas-propellant, and red clover tea is a wonderful digestant.

The heart shares in our joys and sorrows. It expands and contracts with our moods, it weeps with us, grieves with us, moans with us, and it can even injure itself in our excessive joys. It may quiver from the impact of a brainstorm whose vortex uproots the most solid anchorage. We could live longer if we could spare our hearts the responsibilities of partnership in our physical, moral, mental, and emotional enterprises. When the weary and battle-scarred hearts of ordinary people join the countless army of those that have gone before and the numberless legion that will likewise follow, may the rewards of each be commensurate with their sacrifice.

CHAPTER 5

THE REVERSAL PROCESS AND THE HEALING CRISIS

> *A healing crisis is an acute reaction resulting from the ascendancy of Nature's healing forces over disease conditions. Its tendency is toward recovery, and it is, therefore, in conformity with Nature's constructive principle.*"
> —From a catechism of Naturopathy

I would like to discuss what happens after we are well into an elimination and detoxifying program. A healing crisis is the result of an industrious effort by every organ in the body to eliminate waste products and set the stage for regeneration. It conforms with Hering's Law of Cure, which states, "All cure is from the head down, from the inside out, and in reverse order as symptoms first appeared."

Through this constructive progress toward health, old tissues are replaced with new. A disease crisis, on the other hand, is a natural but unfavorable one. Every organ in the body works against it, rather than with it as in the healing crisis. Anything that happens, favorable or unfavorable, is controlled by natural law.

The experience of going through a healing crisis will seem very much like having disease because of reexperiencing disease symptoms from the past, but there is a very important distinction—elimination. In the healing crisis, the elimination is abundant. The bowel movement is natural. All eliminative organs are doing their part. Right up to the time of the crisis, elimination is regular. But in the diseased state, elimination usually stops or is unsatisfactory, which adds to the symptoms. In the healing crisis, the eliminative processes have become more acute because of the abundance of stored-up energy. Whatever catarrh and other forms of waste have been stored in the body are now in a dissolved, free-flowing state, and a cleansing, purifying process is under way.

By bringing in new nutrients, a stronger foundation is provided. And so it is with the body; new tissue replaces the old. In time, the new tissue becomes strong enough to take its place in the various activities of the body. What becomes of the old tissue? It is not absorbed immediately, nor is it eliminated from the body immediately. It is removed through the bloodstream over a period of months in a gradual process of reabsorption and replacement. This process of building up new cellular structure is accomplished by good blood carrying the right nutrients, and through the circulation of the blood where it is needed. The real cure takes place when the new tissue is exchanged for the old.

The crisis can come without warning, but generally you will know it is close at hand by how wonderful you feel. The final day of the eliminative period comes as an explosion, so to speak. The vital force and energies have been turned loose. This explosion comes only when there is power from this new tissue that has come into activity. The old has spent itself, and the new, built from life-giving foods and health-building processes, has grown stronger than the old, abused tissue. Tissue that has been built from poor food and bad living habits will some day have to wrestle with the stronger tissue created from natural foods. It is plain to see which will dominate. That is why we say a crisis is a blessing in disguise. Most persons cannot realize that they have passed through a "knothole," so to speak, with the new now asserting itself.

There are three stages through which a person must pass in getting well. They are the eliminative, the transitional, and the building stages. The crisis usually occurs during the transitional period, which is the time when the new tissue has matured sufficiently to take on the functions of a more perfect body.

A healing crisis usually lasts about three days, starting with a slight pain and discomfort that may become more severe until the point of complete expulsion has been reached. Following this, the pains diminish. If the energy of the patient is low, the crisis sometimes lasts for a week or more. The stronger the vitality and the greater the power of the patient, the more profoundly she or he will be affected by the crisis.

Although there are many paths which lead to a crisis, fasting will bring a patient into the healing crisis quicker than any other method. Fasting alone is not enough, however, for complete recovery from ailments. The chemical elements that are necessary for rebuilding the body and instructions for proper living should be given by the doctor following a fast.

Many times during a fast, a crisis does not occur. If this is the case, a short time on a health-building program will be necessary before the crisis can develop. All conditions must be in its favor—climate and altitude, the right mental attitude, healthful eating habits, and good elimination. Think of the whole body getting into action and correcting conditions.

Although a crisis cannot be brought about without proper diet, or fasting, the best diet in the world is ineffectual if the patient needs corrective exercises. If there is a mental state causing a great deal of irritation or colitis in the bowel, the best colonic will not cure it—nor even the best of any other physical method. Proper diet and a good bowel condition can accomplish a great deal, yet with a heavy catarrhal condition in the body, there may be many small crises to go through before the final one is possible. Everything must be considered and given its proper place in the buildup to a healing crisis.

A lady patient I had been treating for some time was about due for her healing crisis, I thought, when one morning about two o'clock she telephoned to say she was suffering from excruciating pains in the stomach. When I arrived at her home, she was in the process of using a stomach pump. Upon questioning, I discovered that this patient had changed her diet somewhat, but not enough. She had previously asked if she could have pumpernickel bread. Since she was seventy-five years of age, I did not want to make too many drastic changes or omit bread from her diet completely, which I would have done had she been younger. I had agreed to the pumpernickel bread in her diet, therefore, assuming the intake would be moderate. Needless to say, I was surprised to learn that she had been eating a full loaf of bread with each meal—breakfast, lunch, and dinner. Then I realized, of course, that her pain and distress had nothing to do with the healing crisis. The bread eating had slowed down the process.

The iris gives a wonderful check on the patient. If he or she has been following instructions, the evidence will be there. The type of healing crisis we have been discussing, however, is only for certain persons—those who desire to live in accordance with natural laws.

Years ago I put a man, almost blind and with heart trouble, on a regular health routine of diet, exercise, and rest. About three months after starting treatment, I was called to his home. This man was having heart pains. I knew this was a crisis and that he would come through all right. His crisis lasted twelve hours. Almost immediately afterward, he was able to read the newspaper for the first time in years. Later he was able to read fine print, and in about two months he attended a motion picture. His heart condition was not entirely corrected, but the crisis brought him to the stage of eliminating the toxic material from his body, and the building process which followed restored him to fairly good health.

Remember that when the healing crisis is in progress, there is under way an acute stage of what previously occurred during the course of a disease process. While eliminating the trouble, there is a step-by-step retracing of old symptoms as implied by Dr. Constantine Hering in his Law of Cure. In order to get well, the patient must go through the healing crisis. You must expect it, look for it, and work toward it.

A former patient had spent three years traveling to various doctors and sanitariums throughout the country in an effort to obtain the healing of fourteen leg ulcers. These healed in three weeks' time due to her cooperation in taking nothing but a broth made from the tops of vegetables. No crisis occurred during this three-week period, but after about three months under my care, this patient lost her sight for two days.

At first she could not understand why this should happen, and then she remembered an incident a number of years before when, as a piano teacher, she had worked so intensely in preparing for a recital that she lost her sight for two days. After this lapse of time, her sight was restored to the state when the disorder began.

Usually people forget what diseases or injuries they may have had in the past, but during the crisis they are almost always reminded of what they had forgotten.

This same patient I just mentioned had an extreme curvature of the spine. As her healing progressed, she developed a severe "cold" that lasted fifteen or twenty days. It was necessary to assist her reversal process with frequent eliminative treatments. During one of these treatments, she underwent the retracing of an experience she had gone through in an accident fifteen years previously. For a few moments, she seemed to go all to pieces. Her tongue swelled and she could hardly talk. For fifteen minutes or so her body shook all over, and she seemed to be in a critical condition. But after this experience was over, the spinal tension disappeared, the curvature was less, and there was constant improvement in the spine throughout the following year. She felt better than she had in many years.

These case histories are presented because I want to verify the rule that there is a step-by-step retracing, in the reverse order, of the disease conditions experienced through life. The retracing process is justified when we stop to think that a person's living habits and the food he eats determines the kind of tissue he has. In order to rid the body of the tissue built from injurious living habits—tissue that holds disease symptoms latent in chronic tissue—the retracing process, the healing crisis, is necessary. We suffer the sins of our flesh. We suffer during the processes of the healing crisis, which is the final purification process.

We should not force a tissue into an acute condition unless the whole body is ready for it. The eliminative processes of the kidneys will be more active and the results more permanent if the other eliminative organs are functioning more than adequately. The stomach can better overcome its problem if the bowel is working normally. If there is a bronchial discharge and elimination, the bowels will aid in this, the elimination becoming more complete as the patient goes through the crisis. In producing a crisis, as much help as possible is needed from every organ. This is why a healing crisis is more successful when the doctor has been treating the "organism as a whole" rather than only certain organs, as is so often done in ordinary office practice. The doctor who understands the healing crisis knows that it progresses most satisfactorily when a complete right-living program is being followed.

We can almost always predict the approach of a crisis through iridology. We know that when a patient begins to gather strength and seems almost well, we can be assured that the tissues are being supplied with a superabundance of clean, healthy blood. It is this clean, nutrient-rich blood that is going to build healthier tissue and lead the way into the healing crisis. Keeping in mind the conditions just mentioned, doctors should judge when they would expect a healing crisis to appear, and then tell the patient, within a certain number of weeks, when he or she may expect his or her crisis.

You can help to bring out a reaction in any organ of the body through stimulation, and there are many methods that will accomplish this purpose. An organ whose processes have been speeded up will absorb more nourishment, but I have found that stimulation to individual organs does not produce lasting effects. The reason is that there isn't healthy support from the other organs of the body. This is one reason why I do not believe in concentrating treatment on any one organ when the condition requiring correction is constitutional. In a complete healing crisis, for the good of the whole body, every organ manifests changes for the better. In this way, whatever change has come about will remain because the whole structure has been strengthened enough to maintain the revitalized condition.

I am reminded of the case of a man with stomach trouble. After treating him for some time, the stomach condition was cleared up, but during the crisis he developed a very severe backache. When I questioned him, he could not recall having had any backache in the past, but after he completed the crisis he came in to see me. He reported that he remembered a fall from a porch as a child, after which he had the same kind of back pain that he experienced during the crisis.

Another patient was suffering from ulcers of the stomach. From examining his iris, I found that this young man had sulfur deposits in his system, and, although he said he had never taken sulfur into his body, sulfur was there. Upon further questioning, I learned that he had worked in a fruit drying or packing plant where sulfur was used. He had breathed the sulfur into his system. There are many ways of introducing substances into our systems without knowing it, as we see from the example of this young man who inhaled sulfur at work.

At the time of the healing crisis, this patient broke out with a skin rash. We must always expect some kind of skin rash or eruption when there is sulfur in the system. In an experiment conducted at an eastern university, a number of boys were each given ¼ teaspoon of sulfur. Within thirty days, they all broke out with boils.

There is not only the physical healing crisis, but the mental crisis as well. As an example, in one of my cases, the physical improvement that resulted from fasting brought about a tissue response in the brain. I asked the patient whether there was something bothering her and if she would like to talk things over. She replied that there was nothing on her mind.

Two or three days later she asked to talk to me and went into a prolonged crying spell. She unraveled quite a story, telling me she had lost a child because the doctor who delivered the baby was under the influence of liquor at the time. The baby was born dead, and the doctor said it was because she had contracted a disease from her husband (which I later showed her was not true). The story was probably fabricated by the doctor to cover his own guilt. This memory had tormented her for many years, and as a result she had developed an underlying resentment toward her husband and rejection of the sexual act, which had brought about such a painful experience. In my talk with her I cleared up the problem by showing her that she had a distorted conception of what had happened. By pointing out that even if she had a disease, the fast would have overcome it through the healing crisis. I pointed out that there were others who had stillborn babies and had not developed mental complexes, and that it was to her advantage to clear up this mental situation. After our talk she seemed like a new person.

Eventually, she passed through her mental crisis, and after she returned home it was gratifying to receive a letter telling me how happy she was and how her married life had been practically made over because she now knew that her husband bore no fault in the matter.

To have mental fixations and complexes cleared out of the mind is just as important as cleaning out the bowel or any organ structure of the body. In the process of trying to heal people through fasting, you will find that in many cases, a long fast results in a psychic crisis. These psychic crises are difficult to handle, and it takes considerable patience and understanding to carry the patient through. At the time the patient is in a mental state of reviewing the past, he or she will respond only to someone in whom they have complete confidence. The person who is taking care of the patient must be in tune with them emotionally. The patient may divulge many things from his or her subconscious mind that they may deny after the crisis is over. We know there are many memories and problems buried in the mind that can be the cause of serious difficulties. I have heard patients undergoing crisis relate incidents that happened twenty or thirty years previously. Some of them bring up experiences in their sexual past that they would not reveal under other circumstances. This is one of the best housecleaning processes for a patient. However, I do not advise prolonging a fast for the purpose of developing a psychic crisis.

On occasion I have used the assistance of a surgeon in a crisis. One such case was that of a male patient who had an inherent weakness in the right groin with lymphatic involvement. Catarrhal congestion was present throughout the body. As the result of treatment, the catarrhal settlement was being eliminated through the glands in the groin. A swelling the size of a grapefruit formed. It seemed foolish to allow this mass to be absorbed and carried through the body for ultimate elimination, possibly through the lungs, kidneys, and bowels. Without an anesthetic, it was lanced, and a quart and a half of pus was drained out.

Since the patient's body had brought on the crisis, I believe it would have handled this eliminative process, but considering that the groin is not a vital organ, we decided in favor of draining the toxic material out through the skin. If a vital organ, such as the bowel or the kidney, had been involved, we would have left it to be eliminated through the natural channels. The surgeon working with me was an osteopathic physician who knew what a crisis was and understood what I wished to accomplish. The patient's psoriasis also cleared up after the crisis.

No two cases are alike. Because everyone lives life unlike their neighbor's, has a dissimilar occupation, an environment he or she may be subconsciously fighting, an attitude of tension and pressure; there may be fifty different causes leading to fifty different diseases.

During the time of crisis, there is an absence of appetite. One should follow the body's natural cravings. At this time, the body needs water to help carry off the toxins that have reached the elimination point and this is a time for rest. "Rest it out," is an expression I use during the crisis period, and I mean mental as well as physical rest.

The patient should be advised not to overeat during a crisis and to eat foods that will assist the eliminative process. During the height of the crisis, the patient should abstain from eating for the most part, to give the body a chance to work on the healing processes, or eat only a very small quantity of food. Consider the body as being like a bank. If there has been a consistent deposit in the bank during the building process, there will be enough strength to draw upon when needed. If the patient is on a fast at the time the crisis comes, the doctor might have him continue to the next period of seven days before breaking the fast. If he is feeling fine, however, and everything seems to be favorable, the fast may then be broken.

The crisis is not the accomplishment of the doctor, nor that of the patient, directly. The body's processes accomplish it. The intelligence within the patient's body knows more about tissue structure repair and regeneration than any doctor could possibly know, regardless of the system of healing in which he believes.

The crisis time usually is when the doctor does the least for the patient. The effort is wholly expended by the body to normalize itself, and, in most cases, it should be left alone to do this job. The doctor should be alert for fears that may develop, however, and should avoid treatments that either suppress or stimulate elimination. The body that is capable of producing this

---

∽ Important Crisis Note

A crisis comes usually after you feel your best. It is the will of nature. No doctor or patient or food can bring on a crisis. It comes when your body is ready. It does it in its own time. It goes through slow or fast according to the patient's constitution, nervous system, and what you have earned so that it will come on. You *earn* this crisis through hard work. It comes through a sacrifice, giving up bad habits, taking a new path, cleaning up the act that you've been in when your life wasn't working with the laws of nature. A crisis can come harsh, small, violently, or softly, according to what is possible for the body to control and take care of. Some crises come in backaches, skin rashes, joint pains, or teeth can become on edge and diarrhea can develop. I have seen people with all of these symptoms; however, they do not usually come at the same moment but move from one part of the body to another or wherever the body is placing its energy for cleansing, rejuvenation, and getting rid of the old tissue and acids that probably have accumulated over a period of years.

healing is making a normal readjustment and needs no outside help. In most of these cases, it is not what doctors do for the patient but what they do not do that is important.

There does not seem to be the incentive to prevent disease that there should be today, nor do we have adequate education or the health ideals each individual should strive for to carry out his own health program. It is regrettable that some persons are merely interested in getting by and seem unaware that they are committing slow suicide every waking moment. They are not interested in health until they lose it, or until their work is hampered; then they start looking for something to remedy their condition. When such a patient has been given up by his doctors, he at last awakens to the seriousness of his problem and is frightened enough to do something about it. The nature cure doctor often gets this patient when his hope is almost gone.

It is up to the doctors to bring their patients through the crises for a cure, but they should not always promise a cure, because there is no such thing as an absolute cure for everyone. It is for the doctor to decide with the patient just how a condition should be cared for, and the doctor should tell the patient exactly the way he works so he will know what to expect.

Do you see now what I mean by the healing crisis? Relatively little is generally known about it, or written about it, so far. Few doctors know very much about it. I feel fortunate that I have been able to observe all that I have concerning the healing crisis, and I have done my best to analyze and catalogue this information. The body could manifest no greater proof of its ability to be self-adjusting, self-regenerating, and self-healing than it does through the retracing of disease and the production of a healing crisis.

CHAPTER 6

FOLLOW UP WITH A BALANCED FOOD REGIMEN

Following a healing crisis or completion of an elimination diet regimen or fast, it is essential to turn to a right way of eating, a "nondiet" so to speak. We all need to work toward a fully nourishing, toxin-free food regimen that provides all the right nutrients for building new tissue while promoting adequate elimination of normal wastes and toxins from both internal processes and the external environment. Over the years I have developed what I call my "Health and Harmony Food Regimen," and in this chapter I am going to introduce you to it. But first, I need to share a fact of life with you.

A healthy food regimen may (and nearly always does) include foods that you don't like. Nevertheless, it is my experience that we can learn to like such foods by setting our minds to like them. I didn't used to like avocados or broccoli, but because I know my body needs them, I like them. You can do the same. Almost everyone can name several foods they like now but didn't used to like. So, make up your mind that you are going to learn to like foods that are good for you. Usually, vegetables are the big challenge in this regard, and often the key to enjoying vegetables is to find seasonings and salad dressings that make them taste great. Go to your local health food store and ask for suggestions. Personally, I like to sprinkle my own brand of broth powder on my vegetables. It tastes great even without salt. (Sometimes I use a little natural sea salt.)

I want you to face reality in another regard. The best food regimen in the world cannot keep you healthy if you persist in destructive lifestyle habits. Get rid of the cigarettes, the drugs, the alcohol, the sweets, the coffee, the sodas—and anything else that you know you do in excess. If that brings out a groan in you, just realize that if thousands of others have done it, so can you. Once you have tasted the joy and freedom of living a healthy life, you will find a greater satisfaction in your work, relationships, hobbies, and even in your various other responsibilities. You won't want to go back to the old life.

When I was young, I almost died from a diet that consisted completely of foods that tasted wonderful—Danish pastry, milk shakes, fried foods, and lots of desserts. I developed a dangerous lung infection called bronchiectasis. That was in the days before antibiotics, and the only advice my doctor could suggest was bed rest. A Seventh-Day Adventist doctor changed my life by giving me a crash course in health-building foods. He introduced me to salads, which I had steered away from previously. I wanted to get well so badly that I changed my way of eating, and I began breathing exercises in earnest. I gave up sweets and health-destructive treats. It took nearly a year, but I got rid of that infection and I am now ninety-two years of age at the time of this writing.

Most Americans develop food preferences from their family food patterns, and when kids grow up they tend to prefer what they liked at home. Newly married wives often cater to their husbands' preferences by learning to cook what the husband likes. Such thoughtless practices are often in conflict with the wonderful food and nutrition knowledge that has been gathered by nutritionists, biochemists, microbiologists, and other researchers.

Most people eat too much red meat, milk products, wheat products, and sugar-rich foods. Too much meat causes putrefaction in the bowel. Too many milk products slow bowel transit time, encourage constipation, and bring on catarrh. Too many wheat products (especially those made with refined white flour) can damage bowel walls, slow bowel transit time, lead to weight gain, and stimulate lots of catarrh. Too many sugary foods cause increased fat intake and storage, contribute to bowel fermentation, feed undesirable bowel bacteria, and overwhelm the pancreas (islets of Langerhans, insulin release sites). Over 50 percent of the American people are obese because of ignorance about foods, fat-depositing meals, and lack of exercise.

To start your new food regimen, clean out your cupboards and pantry. Get rid of the foods that cause problems and restock with foods you'll need in order to follow my Health and Harmony Food Regimen. Get rid of refined carbohydrates and substitute honey, molasses, and dried fruits for sugar (nonsugar artificial sweeteners may be dangerous to your health), and trade refined flour for whole grain products. For milk products, substitute soy milk and tofu, raw seed and nut milks and butters, sorbets, and goat milk cheeses. Occasional use of yogurt, kefir, and clabbered milk is okay.

My regimen requires that you avoid fatty meats and use lean red meats only a few times monthly. Switch to mostly poultry and fish, and the fish should have white meat, fins, and scales (salmon is okay too). Broil, bake, or steam meat, fish, and poultry; don't fry anything, and don't cook with meat fat or concentrated vegetable oils. (I recommend that you throw away your frying pans.) Use meat, fish, and poultry only three times weekly, substituting vegetarian meals and proteins other than meat on all other days. Cheese, tofu, yogurt, and beans are all good proteins.

Avoid caffeinated drinks and sodas high in phosphates. Caffeine overstimulates the nerves, interferes with glucose metabolism, and is hard on the bowel wall. High-phosphate sodas leech calcium out of the body as the phosphate is excreted in the urine. Herbal teas and natural coffee substitutes are better for you, and fruit juices are health-building while sodas are not. Keep in mind that decaffeinated coffee still has 2 percent of its caffeine left.

Table salt (sodium chloride) is refined at high temperatures and is a refined product, not a natural food. Many Americans eat several times the RDI (reference daily intake) of 2.4 grams for sodium. It acts more like a drug in the body than a food and is a risk factor for high blood pressure. Instead of so much salt, use herbal seasonings, spices, and broth powder for seasoning. As a matter of fact, we get all the sodium we need from the food we eat. But, if you have to have salt for flavoring, use a little sea salt, in which sodium chloride is balanced with other mineral salts.

Use as much fresh produce as you can, and use canned or packaged foods only as a last resort. Fresh fruit and vegetables have more food value than any other form, whether canned, dried, or stored in a dark, cool cellar. You get not only vitamins, minerals, live enzymes, a little protein, and lots of complex carbohydrates from veggies and fruits, but you also get fiber, which is needed to carry off cholesterol, triglycerides, and a certain amount of toxins as well as normalizing bowel transit time. (I would call fiber an elimination food because of its cleansing effect; chlorophyll is also a cleansing food.)

How many different fresh fruits and vegetables do you eat in a week? Can you write them down from memory? Think about the last time you shopped in the produce section of your favorite market and see how many of the fresh fruits and vegetables you can name that you don't usually eat. Do they outnumber those that you usually buy? I challenge you to buy two new vegetables or fruits next week that you've never eaten before and try them out. Then buy and try two more the week after, and keep doing it until you've tried everything in the produce section of the store.

I believe the best fruits and vegetables are those grown in organic, mineral-rich, uncontaminated soils. It is possible for foods labeled "organic" to be grown on mineral deficient soil, so don't take for granted that every food labeled "organic" has all the nutrients it should have.

Iceberg lettuce is almost nutrionally worthless, so don't waste your money. Other kinds of lettuce have much more chlorophyll, vitamins, minerals, and overall food value. Most citrus is picked green for shipping purposes, so I don't recommend it. If you can get tree-ripened citrus, buy it and eat it—sliced in sections—for the fiber and vitamin C. We get our natural B-complex vitamins from fruit and vegetables, excepting B_{12}, which is mostly found in animal products. Sometimes there are traces of vitamin B_{12} in vegetables grown on soil enriched with animal manure, but you can't be sure. I have read that B_{12} is found in spirulina (an edible alga with great and varied nutritional value). I think it is not assimilated as well in comparison with meat and dairy sources of this vitamin.

Throw out most if not all of your canned and packaged foods and anything else that has been processed, packaged, or adulterated with chemical additives. Processing always reduces food value and increases price. Most contain sugar and salt, sometimes more additives. They are all lower in nutritional value than fresh foods.

Those who have read ancient history books know that foraging, hunting, and fishing were typical of early human survival. Agricultural and domestic livestock came later. In the earliest days, man lived close to nature, using only whole, pure, natural, and fresh foods. Our bodies were adapted to such food sources and, as I see it, fresh, raw, natural foods are more compatible to our bodies than anything else.

FOOD LAWS TO FOLLOW

1. Daily Diet

Daily diet should be 80 percent alkaline and 20 percent acid foods, as shown in Table 6.1 on page 82. This means that you should select eight alkaline foods and two acid foods daily.

2. Natural

Fifty percent to 60 percent of the food eaten should be raw. If, for any reason, you can't follow this law, take 1 teaspoon of wheat bran or psyllium husks after each meal. This will take care of the fiber needed in your diet.

3. Proportion

Eat six vegetables, two fruits, one starch, and one protein daily. (This keeps your daily food total 80 percent alkaline, 20 percent acid.) This balance matches what the blood should be.

4. Variety

Vary proteins, starches, vegetables, and fruits from meal to meal and day to day. Know seven good proteins, seven good starches, seven good salad dressings, and seven herb teas so you get variety.

5. Excess

Excess in one or a few foods is to be avoided because this creates imbalance in the body. Wheat, milk, and sugar are the greatest offenders I know, and they all contribute to weight problems. Excess eating of all foods, even in a balanced eating regimen, leads to the development of fatty tissue, a condition of imbalance within the body. Any form of excess leads to an imbalance of some kind.

6. Deficiency

Deficiency in foods containing the chemical elements, vitamins, and other nutrients causes imbalance in the body and, in general, prevents tissue repair and rebuilding. This is especially important with regard to inherently weak organs of the body, which are unable to hold nutrients and chemical elements as well as normal tissues. The most common deficiencies I have encountered are calcium, sodium, silicon, and iodine, and these should be obtained from foods or supplements derived from foods.

7. Combinations

Separate proteins and starches: one at lunch, one at dinner. Have fruit for breakfast and, if desired, at 3:00 P.M. If reducing, have two protein meals and only one starch meal in the regular regimen.

Table 6.1. **Acid–Alkaline Food**

Nonstarch Foods

AL Alfalfa	AL Endive
AL Artichokes	AL Garlic
AL Asparagus	AL Horseradish
AL Beans (string)	AL Kale
AL Beans (wax)	AL Kohlrabi
AL Beet leaves	AL Leeks
AL Beets (whole)	AL Lettuce
AL Broccoli	AL Mushrooms
AL Cabbage (red)	AL Okra
AL Cabbage (white)	AL Olives (ripe)
AL Carrot tops	AL Onions
AL Carrots	AL Osterplant
AL Cauliflower	AL Parsley
AL Celery knobs	AL Parsnips
AL Chickory	AL Peas (fresh)
AL Coconut	AL Peppers (sweet)
AL Corn	AL Radishes
AL Cucumbers	AL Rutabagas
AL Dandelions	AL Savory
AL Eggplant	AL Sea lettuce

AL Sorrel
AL Soybean products
AL Spinach
AL Sprouts
AL Summer squash
AL Swiss chard
AL Turnips
AL Watercress

Proteins and Fruits

AL Apples
AL Apricots
AL Avocados
AC Beef
AL Berries (all)
AC Buttermilk
AL Cantaloupes
AC Chicken
AC Clams
AC Cottage cheese
AC Crab
AL Cranberries
AL Currants
AL Dates
AC Duck
AC Eggs
AL Figs
AC Fish
AC Goose
AL Grapes
AL Honey (pure)
AC Jell-O

AC Lamb
AL Lemons
AL Limes
AC Lobster
AC Mutton
AC Nuts
AL Oranges
AC Oysters
AL Peaches
AL Pears
AL Persimmons
AL Pineapple
AL Plums
AC Pork
AL Prunes
AC Rabbit
AL Raisins
AC Raw sugar
AL Rhubarb
AL Tomatoes
AC Turkey
AC Turtle
AC Veal

Starchy Foods

AL Bananas
AC Barley
AC Beans (lima)
AC Beans (white)
AC Breads
AC Cereals
AC Chestnuts

(Continued)

Table 6.1. **Continued**

AC Corn	AC Peas (dried)
AC Cornmeal	AC Potatoes (sweet)
AC Cornstarch	AL Potatoes (white)
AC Crackers	AL Pumpkin
AC Gluten flour	AC Rice (brown)
AC Grapefruit	AC Rice (polished)
AC Lentils	AC Rye
AC Macaroni	AC Rye flour
AC Maize	AC Sauerkraut
AC Millet	AL Squash (Hubbard)
AC Oatmeal	AC Tapioca
AC Peanut butter	AC Whole wheat
AC Peanuts	

Source: Ragnar Berg of Germany.

Note: Foods preceded by the letters AL are alkaline forming; foods preceded by the letters AC are acid forming.

8. Cooking

Cook with low heat, without water, or with only a little water in waterless cookware with the lid left on. Don't peek; leave the lid on until done to avoid air exposure to hot food. Waterless cooking at 185°F destroys only 2 percent of nutrients, as compared to 20 percent in steaming (212°F) and 50 percent in boiling foods. Use unsprayed vegetables, if available, and prepare them as soon after picking as possible. Steaming, of course, is preferable to boiling.

9. Bake, Broil, or Roast

If meat is used, choose lean meat—no fat, no pork. Never fry or cook in heated oils.

It is important for us to realize that we should take more of our foods on the raw side, which is not as fattening and has the advantage of providing more live enzymes to help the body use its nutrients better. Raw vegetables in a salad are wonderful for us. We can even use raw asparagus, squash, and spinach in salads.

We can put raw foods in a liquefier and have blended fruit or vegetable drinks. I call them health cocktails. Of course, we must be careful about adding cream or butter.

Most people eat too many acid-forming foods: meat, eggs, milk, wheat products, and starchy foods. As we have mentioned, a government survey has shown that 56 percent of the average American diet is made up of wheat and milk products. These are the greatest weight builders when taken in excess. These foods should only be 6 percent of the American diet. We need to eat more fresh vegetables and fruits with our meals. In doing this, we reduce taking in too many starches and proteins, and we produce a better acid/alkaline balance.

Whole grains, vegetables, and fruits (complex carbohydrates) not only supply a steady flow of glucose to energize the cells of the body, but they provide vitamins and minerals needed by the thousands of enzymes in the body to activate cellular processes essential to life and physical activity. They also supply fiber, which is necessary for colon health. A recent survey showed that the average person in this country only takes in 7 grams of fiber for every 1,000 calories of food, and that is very low. A survey by the Archway Company showed that 76 percent of the people interviewed knew that fiber was important in the diet, but 99 percent didn't know how much daily soluble fiber they needed. Only 55 percent could name good sources of fiber. An article in the *Journal of the American Medical Association* in 1996 said that every 10-gram increase in daily fiber intake lowers the risk of heart attack by 30 percent.

The American Dietetic Association recommends at least 20 to 25 grams of fiber daily.

When my health ranch was running at its peak, I instructed all our cooks to follow the principle of using whole, pure, and natural foods in a half-building, half-eliminating food regimen. Of course, I used reducing diets for those who requested them, but my regular Health and Harmony Food Regimen was what I call a maintenance food program, one that people could use for the rest of their lives to cultivate the best of health. Before I present some sample menus, here are some daily tips to follow.

Upon arising, drink a large cup of hot water with a teaspoon of liquid chlorophyll in it. Many people find that this aids in stimulating a healthy, comfortable bowel movement. You may want to schedule your morning skin brushing at this time. Then, about a half hour before breakfast, take a glass of fruit juice, such as grape, pineapple, prune, apple, kiwi-strawberry, or black cherry. A cup of hot broth or a lecithin drink may be taken instead. Add 1 tablespoon vegetable broth powder and/or 1 tablespoon lecithin granules to a glass of warm water. Herbal teas are also recommended.

Between juice or drink and breakfast, I suggest that you skin brush for two to five minutes, exercise on a mini-trampoline to music, take a walk in a garden or a short hike, or do other exercises.

BREAKFAST

Have fresh fruit, a health drink, and one starch; or two fruits, one protein, and a health drink; or fruit only. Soak dried fruits, such as unsulfured apricots, prunes, figs, apples, or pears in boiling water for five minutes before using. Fresh fruit of any kind may be used—melons, grapes, peaches, pears, berries, or apples. Use fruit in season when possible; don't eat melons and sour fruit together. Sprinkle baked or stewed fruit with ground nuts or nut butter, especially sesame nut butter.

The following menus are adapted from instructions to the kitchen staff members when my sanitarium at the ranch was in full swing.

Fruit

One fresh fruit and one dried fruit. For reducing, cut down on dried fruits. Prunes have a lot of fiber.

Drinks

Raw nut or seed milk, soy milk, or rice milk, if desired; whey; and tea (three different kinds of teas should be served during the day; five different kinds should be kept on hand in the kitchen).

Cereals

Always serve five different kinds during the week: Yellow corn-meal (twice a week), muesli (twice a week), rye, brown rice, and millet. Whole grain cereal should be cooked over very low heat, tightly covered; use double boiler or soak overnight in boiling water in a wide-mouth thermos.

Supplements

For sprinkling on cereals or fruits: Wheat germ, rice polishings, flaxseed meal, and sesame seed meal.

Eggs

Soft- and hard-boiled or poached.

Sunday Mornings

It's okay to serve cornmeal hot cakes with honey or pure maple syrup.

Coffee Substitutes

Any of the toasted grain or vegetable-based products.

10 A.M.

Juice time—vegetable or fruit; or substitute vegetable broth.

SUGGESTED BREAKFAST MENUS

Monday
Fresh fruit
Reconstituted dried apricots
Millet
Supplements
Oat straw tea
(Add eggs or cottage cheese for protein)

Tuesday
Fresh figs
Cornmeal cereal
Supplements
Shave grass tea
(Add eggs or nut butter, if desired,
or raw applesauce and blackberries)

or
Coddled egg, supplements, and herb tea

Wednesday
Fresh fruit
Reconstituted dried peaches
Millet cereal
Supplements
Add eggs or cheese for protein
Alfalfa tea

Thursday
Fresh fruit
Reconstituted prunes
Brown rice (cold or warm) with raisins,
cinnamon, sunflower seeds, honey
For protein, yogurt with fruit and nut butter
Supplements
Herb tea

Friday
Slices of fresh pineapple with shredded coconut
Buckwheat cereal
Supplements
Peppermint tea
or
Baked apple, persimmons, chopped raw almonds,
acidophilus milk, supplements, and herb tea

Saturday
Muesli with bananas, dates, and seed-, nut-, or rice milk
Supplements
Dandelion coffee or herb tea

Sunday
Cooked applesauce with raisins
Rye cereal
Supplements
Shave grass tea
or
Cantaloupe and strawberries, cottage cheese,
supplements, and herb tea

When starting out with a new diet or eating regimen, it is best for the cook to allow the family a transition time to get used to the changes. Rushing people or trying to force them breeds counterproductive results. So, be patient.

The basics of this daily food regimen are two different fruits, six or more vegetables, one protein, and one starch, using fruit or vegetable juices or herb teas as between-meal snacks. Chlorophyll tea (1 teaspoon liquid chlorophyll in 1 cup of hot water) can be used in place of fruit juice. Use at least two green leafy vegetables every day. I advise that 50 to 60 percent of the total intake be raw food. Isn't that easy to remember?

LUNCH

Salad Bar

Always serve: Finely shredded carrots, beets, turnips, carrot sticks, celery sticks, sliced tomatoes, sliced cucumbers, sliced green peppers, and alfalfa sprouts (other sprouts may be served occasionally).

Anything else in season, used raw: Jicama, zucchini, summer squash, onions (small), parsley, watercress, endive.

Twice a week: Stuffed celery (with almond or cashew butter).

Once or twice a week: Olives, Waldorf salad (peel apples), gelatin mold (with shredded carrots and pineapple).

Once a week: Carrot and pea salad with cheese, cole slaw, carrot and cashew salad (made with a Champion juicer), stuffed dates (almond or cashew butter).

Salad dressings: Using mashed avocado, yogurt, or nut butter as a base, add cottage cheese, blue cheese, Romano cheese, or Parmesan cheese together with your favorite herbal seasonings. Traditional oil and vinegar with a little honey is always acceptable. Use as little dressing as possible—a tablespoon or two—to avoid excess calories.

Vegetables

Two, cooked. Use one grown under the ground and one grown above the ground. One bland vegetable must be served, such as beets, squash (yellow neck, banana, winter, etc.), zucchini, peas, carrots, string beans, wax beans, spinach, or asparagus. Other vegetables may include a sulfur type (doesn't have to), such as cabbage, cauliflower, brussels sprouts, onions, broccoli, turnips, or kohlrabi. Steamed onions may be served (creamed with parsley) once a week, as a separate dish.

Starches

Brown rice (twice a week), baked potato (twice a week), lima beans, cornbread, yams.

The four best starches are yellow cornmeal, rye, brown rice, and millet. Other starches include barley (winter starch), buckwheat, baked or dead ripe banana, winter squash, baked potato, and baked sweet potato. For variety, include steel-cut oatmeal, whole wheat cereal, Shredded Wheat, rye crackers, bran muffins, bread (whole grain, rye, soy, cornbread, and bran breads are preferred).

Drinks

The best health drinks are vegetable broth, soup, coffee substitutes, buttermilk, raw milk, goat's milk, rice milk, soy milk, raw nut or seed milk, oat straw tea, alfalfa-mint tea, huckleberry tea, mint tea, whey, carrot juice, V-8 juice, or any health drink. Water is often the most needed health drink, especially for the elderly.

Vegetarians

Use soybeans, lima beans, cottage cheese, sunflower seeds, and other seeds; also seed butters, nut butters, nut milk drinks, tofu, and eggs. Use meat substitutes or vegetarian proteins.

Twice a week: Low-fat cottage cheese or any cheese that breaks, such as roquefort, blue cheese, or feta.

Once a week: Egg omelet. If you have a protein at this meal, a health dessert is allowed but not recommended. Avoid eating proteins and starches together. They are deliberately separated on all meal plans so that you will eat more vegetables. The noon meal may be exchanged for the evening meal, provided the same regimen is upheld. Exercise is necessary to handle raw food; generally, more exercise is good after the noon meal. Sandwiches, if eaten, should be combined with vegetables at the same meal.

SUGGESTED LUNCH MENUS

Monday
Vegetable salad
Baby lima beans
Baked potato
Spearmint tea

Tuesday
Vegetable salad with health mayonnaise
Steamed asparagus
Very ripe bananas
or
Steamed unpolished brown rice
Vegetable broth or herb tea

Wednesday
Raw salad plate with sour cream dressing
Cooked green beans
Cornbread and/or baked Hubbard squash
Sassafras tea

Thursday
Salad with French dressing
Baked zucchini and okra
Corn on the cob
Ry-Krisp
Buttermilk or herb tea

Friday

Salad

Baked green peppers stuffed with eggplant and tomatoes

Baked potato and/or bran muffin

Carrot soup or herb tea

Saturday

Salad

Turnips and turnip greens

Baked yam

Catnip tea

Sunday

Salad with lemon and olive oil dressing

Steamed whole barley

Cream of celery soup

Steamed chard

Herb tea

DINNER

Protein

Meat (lean; no fat, no pork), such as chicken, turkey, meat loaf, lamb roast. A meat meal is to be served three times a week.

Fish

Have fish at least one day a week. Baked fish, such as ocean white fish, halibut, bass, trout, and salmon loaf, are good. Fresh salmon and canned sardines are very high in RNA (ribonucleic acid) for tissue rebuilding.

Vegetables

Have two cooked vegetables and salad, as for lunch.

Fruit and Cheese

Two nights a week, have three kinds of assorted fresh fruit, such as melons, apples, persimmons, pears, cherries, berries, oranges, apricots, peaches, nuts, or dates. Have assorted cheeses, such as Swiss, jack, cheddar, cottage cheese. Yogurt is also a good option. Crackers, such as Ry-Krisp, Ak-Mak, or sesame, can be included.

Juices

It is all right to have a juice in place of any meal. Those on juice diets should have juice every three hours as follows: 8 A.M.—fruit juice; 11 A.M.—carrot juice; 2 P.M.—carrot juice; 5 P.M.—fruit juice.

Vegetarians

Nut loaf is a good protein option for vegetarians. Cheese soufflé, cottage cheese loaf, and eggplant and cheese loaf are great cheese options.

SUGGESTED DINNER MENUS

Monday
Salad
Diced celery and carrots
Steamed spinach (waterless-cooked)
Puffy omelet
Vegetable broth

Tuesday

Salad

Cooked beet tops

Broiled steak or ground beef patties

Cauliflower

Comfrey tea

Wednesday

Cottage cheese

Cheese sticks

Apples, peaches, grapes, nuts

Apple concentrate cocktail

Thursday

Salad

Steamed chard

Baked eggplant

Grilled liver and onions

Persimmon whip (optional)

Alfalfa-mint tea

Friday

Salad with yogurt and lemon dressing

Steamed mixed greens

Beets

Steamed fish (with lemon slices)

Leek soup

Saturday

Salad

Cooked string beans

Baked summer squash

Carrot and cheese loaf

Cream of lentil soup or lemongrass tea
Fresh peach gelatin
Almond nut cream

Sunday
Salad
Diced carrots and peas
Steamed tomato aspic
Roast leg of lamb
Mint tea

MENU EXCHANGES

If the noon and evening meals are exchanged, follow the same regimen. Starches make you sleepy; proteins are stimulating. If insomnia is a problem, meals may be switched for better results. Starch meals are for physical labor; proteins for mental work.

Never eat when emotionally upset, chilled, overtired, overheated, ill, or lacking the keenest desire for the simplest food.

Missing a meal will do you more good. Some may want to have an extra juice about 8:00 P.M.

Fruit juice may be apple, grape, papaya, or liquid chlorophyll (½ to 1 teaspoon to an 8-ounce glass of water). Liquid chlorophyll may be used at 8 P.M. instead of juice. Those trying to lose weight can substitute a chlorophyll and water drink for any fruit or fruit juice.

Desserts: Always allowed on Sunday and two other times a week. Gelatin mold (cherry, grape, raspberry—two times a week), homemade ice cream (frozen fruit, whey, and honey), carrot cake, custard, apple brown Betty, or yogurt with fresh fruit.

Avoid: All fried foods, foods cooked in hot oil, peanuts, peanut butter, sausage, salami, white flour products, sugar and sugar-rich foods, pickled foods, salted foods, table salt, dips, chocolate, and milk-containing products.

SUPPLEMENTS

Most people who have subsisted a number of years on poor diets find that they are short of biochemical elements. They have lived on devitaminized, demineralized foodstuffs. For this reason, we recommend several supplements for rebuilding and revitalizing. They are not necessary for the person who has been living correctly, not burning up chemical elements faster than they can be replaced, under normal circumstances, and under the proper diet. These supplements are needed to make up what we especially lack in the "average" American diet.

Supplements should be used daily in the diet and served at the dining table. They help counteract the shortages found in the common diet today. Also add them to liquefied drinks, salads, or even desserts.

Acidophilus culture: *Lactobacilus acidophilus* in capsule or liquid form aids in controlling undesirable bowel bacteria, reducing putrefaction, and keeping the bowel clean.

Alfalfa tablets: Alfalfa, rich in chlorophyll and fiber, helps maintain bowel health through the natural cleansing action of chlorophyll and quickened bowel transit time from the fiber.

Beet tablets: Good for sluggish liver and gallbladder, this supplement gently stimulates bowel regularity.

Bee pollen: Rich in lecithin, bee pollen is 20 percent protein and contains all known essential vitamins, twelve essential minerals and trace elements, bioflavonoids, enzymes, complex sugars, plant steroids, and ten fatty acids. Bee pollen increases stamina and quickens recovery time from athletic exertion or physical labor.

Blackstrap molasses (unsulfured): If you can find a health food store that has it, buy it. Molasses is the "residue" from processing sugar beets and sugar cane into pure granulated sugar (sucrose). It is loaded with vitamins and minerals. You can take it straight by the spoonful or add it to other foods. (Not all molasses in the markets is the real thing. Always read the labels.)

Brewer's yeast: A great natural source of B-complex (except B_{12}) and other vitamins, brewer's yeast is high in amino acids and minerals. Because it is high in phosphorus (which requires calcium for balance), brewer's yeast should always be taken with a generous helping of yogurt or other high-calcium food.

Carob: Chocolate-flavored powder made from finely ground legume pods from carob trees. Carob is more nutritious than cocoa and has no caffeine.

Chlorophyll: This wonderful natural cleanser is rich in magnesium and is in all green vegetables, especially the leafy vegetables. It is available in liquid form in health food stores and is very high in the edible algae spirulina and chlorella.

Chlorella: This is a very popular supplement in Asian countries. Chlorella is an edible alga loaded with nutrients and especially noted for a complex protein growth factor that aids in healing damaged tissues. It helps rid the body of heavy metals and other toxins. Chlorella supports the liver and enhances the immune system.

Cod liver oil: Still the all-around best source of vitamins A and D.

Dulse: I recommend Nova Scotia dulse, but if you can't find it, any dulse will supply iodine for the thyroid gland.

Flaxseed (meal): Flaxseed contains omega-3 fatty acids and is the best vegetarian source of fiber. It should be kept refrigerated. Grind it finely and add a little (I mean "a little," like half a teaspoon) to fruit and vegetable juices. Too much will cause the juice to thicken. (It can also be sprinkled on hot or cold cereal.) Omega-3 fatty acids help protect people from heart attacks, and the fiber not only quickens bowel transit time but carries off cholesterol and triglycerides that would normally be assimilated from the bowel into the lymph.

Ginseng: Chinese herbalists regard ginseng (powdered ginseng root) as one of the best (if not the very best) all-around, health-supporting "tonics." It is most effective in the form of tea. Many ginseng users believe it enhances their sex life. I believe *anything* that enhances your health will enhance your sex life.

Herb teas: Fenugreek, comfrey, peppermint, lemongrass, spearmint, chamomile, oat straw (you have to boil this one for five minutes), and red raspberry are all wonderful herb teas. Visit the tea section of your supermarket and check out the variety of herb teas they now carry.

Milk substitutes: The variety of healthy, nutrient-rich substitutes for cow's milk is growing and includes raw nut and seed milks, soy milk, and rice milk.

Niacin: Taking a gram of this B-complex vitamin with every meal can cut down the liver's production of cholesterol and bring blood to the head, improving oxygen supply to the brain. If you want to try it, start with 100 milligrams of niacin to see how well you tolerate the upper body and facial flush that comes with it. Increase by 100 milligrams more each week until you are taking 1,000 milligrams (1 gram) with each meal. Consult your doctor before you try it.

Oat bran: Oat bran offers soluble and insoluble fiber, which shortens bowel transit time and reduces blood levels of tryglycerides and cholesterol. You can sprinkle it on your cereal, salads, or soups; add it to bread, muffin, or bagel recipes; or just take a tablespoonful three times a day or so.

Omega-3 fatty acids: You can get them from eating fish or flaxseed oil. Eskimos survive on a high-fat diet but have a very low incidence of heart disease because they get a lot of omega-3 oils by eating a lot of fish. You can do the same by using flaxseed oil.

Rice bran syrup: Similar to molasses, this syrup adds a great flavor to goat milk, rice or soy milk, and raw nut or seed milk. It is loaded with vitamins and minerals, especially silicon.

Rice polishings (same as bran): Same nutrients as rice bran syrup but not as nutrient dense.

RNA (ribonucleic acid): This specialized nucleic acid is called "the long-life factor," and is found most abundantly in chlorella, canned sardines, and brewer's yeast.

Spirulina: An edible alga harvested from lakes in Latin America and in Africa, spirulina is high in chlorophyll and B-complex vitamins. Some is being grown commercially in the United States under controlled conditions to produce the most nutrient-rich spirulina possible.

Wheat germ/wheat germ oil: Best natural source of vitamin E for fighting free radicals, energy production, and protecting pituitary and adrenal hormones.

Whey: Goat milk whey is one of the best sources of bioorganic sodium and potassium I have ever found, not to mention that it carries a handful of essential minerals or trace elements.

Supplements don't have to be in pill form. A person has to be in good health to assimilate "pill" form supplements. The supplements just discussed can be assimilated by anyone, even though they are concentrated. Use them in cereals, tonics, drinks, dressings, and almost any recipe. However, heat and baking break down lecithin, many vitamins, and minerals.

MORE HELPFUL FOOD AND MEALTIME TIPS

Because you are unique, there are most probably specific ways to enhance your weight-loss program that will work very well for you but not necessarily well for others. The reverse is also true. Don't get too excited when a friend "shares" some great new dieting or weight-loss rumor from the grapevine at a family fitness center, aerobics class, or health food store. Be open-minded but be very cautious.

One tip that has helped many people is to take four capsules or tablets of chlorella or spirulina half an hour before mealtime. Another is to take a heaping teaspoon of bee pollen fifteen minutes before eating. Either one may reduce your appetite.

Apple cider vinegar and honey in a glass of water has helped some individuals lose weight. Add 1 tablespoon of apple cider vinegar and ½ teaspoon of honey to 16 ounces of water. Take this morning and evening.

Limit your fat intake to what you get in foods such as avocado, eggs, and nut and seed butters. Be careful with salad dressings; most are very high in calories.

Make sure you are getting enough iodine to keep your metabolism up and enough vitamin E to help get more oxygen to the brain. Use at least half a teaspoon of dulse flakes every day, or a dulse tablet with morning and evening meals. People under forty should take 400 units of vitamin E per day, and people over forty should increase that to 800 units. If you are using wheat germ oil, you don't need the vitamin E. There is vitamin E in the wheat germ oil.

You may want to use niacin to flush the toxins from organs and peripheral tissues, speed up the elimination process, and reduce production of cholesterol by the liver. Start with 100 milligrams at each meal and work up to 500 milligrams. From 100 to 500 milligrams, add 50 milligrams to the 100 milligrams every four days until you are taking a total of 500 milligrams.

Niacin is vitamin B_3, perfectly safe but uncomfortable to some because of the release of histamines that cause the face, ears, and neck to redden and tingle for fifteen minutes to half an hour. The histaminic response is accompanied by a flushing of blood capillaries and increased circulation.

DR. JENSEN'S EXTREME HUNGER SNACK

I call this my *Special Slim Shake,* and it can be used as a substitute for one or two meals each day because it is such a great building food, with only about half as many calories as a diet meal.

SPECIAL SLIM SHAKE RECIPE
(185 calories)

1 tablespoon skim milk powder, soy powder, whey, or nut powder
1 tablespoon bee pollen
1 teaspoon chlorella granules or 6 tablets
1 sliver avocado or ½ banana
1 cup apple juice or 1½ tablespoons apple concentrate in 1 cup of water

Combine ingredients in blender and blend for 1 minute. Whey can be substituted for the skim milk powder to help develop the friendly bowel flora. This formula builds the red blood cell count; keeps up the blood sugar level; supplies trace elements; provides amino acids, fatty acids, and fiber; and is high in chlorophyll for cleansing the tissues.

GLOSSARY

Catarrh, phlegm, and **mucus** help rid the body of toxic materials, acids, and debris that are harmful to the tissues. The accumulated toxic materials can be eliminated through any orifice and/or through the eliminative channels.

Detoxification relates to the reduction of toxic materials in the body and makes this toxic material easier to eliminate. The first part of my health program involves enabling the body to reject accumulated toxic wastes collected over the years from bad diets and poor health habits.

Elimination and **Elimination diets** relate to discharge from the body of indigestible materials and waste products, which is done through five eliminative organs: skin, kidneys, liver, lungs, and bowel, and we could add another—the lymphatic system.

Healing crisis is a natural consequence of faithfully following the reversal process. It is an effort on the part of all organs to throw off toxic wastes and develop clean, new tissue in place of the old. Though it may seem like a disease crisis, it will not last more than a week or so. It will bring about renewed health.

Reversal process is the retracing of the stages or steps of each disease a person has had, reactivating each one and processing it. Many people who have suppressed diseases all their lives think an elimination process, such as a cold or flu, is a sickness instead of a healing process.

INDEX

9780071836760